Noncommunicable Diseases
in the Developing World

Noncommunicable Diseases in the Developing World

Addressing Gaps in Global Policy and Research

Edited by
Louis Galambos
and
Jeffrey L. Sturchio
with Rachel Calvin Whitehead

Johns Hopkins University Press
Baltimore

© 2014 Johns Hopkins University Press
All rights reserved. Published 2014
Printed in the United States of America on acid-free paper
9   8   7   6   5   4   3   2   1

Johns Hopkins University Press
2715 North Charles Street
Baltimore, Maryland 21218-4363
www.press.jhu.edu

Library of Congress Cataloging-in-Publication Data

Noncommunicable diseases in the developing world : addressing gaps
in global policy and research / edited by Louis Galambos and Jeffrey L.
Sturchio with Rachel Calvin Whitehead.
      p. ; cm.
   Includes bibliographical references and index.
   ISBN-13: 978-1-4214-1292-4 (pbk. : alk. paper)
   ISBN-10: 1-4214-1292-6 (pbk. : alk. paper)
   ISBN-13: 978-1-4214-1293-1 (electronic)
   ISBN-10: 1-4214-1293-4 (electronic)
   I. Galambos, Louis, editor of compilation   II. Sturchio, Jeffrey L.
(Jeffrey Louis), 1952– editor of compilation.   III. Whitehead, Rachel
Calvin, editor of compilation   [DNLM: 1. Chronic Disease—prevention &
control.   2. Chronic Disease—drug therapy.   3. Developing Countries.
4. Health Policy.   5. Health Services Accessibility.   WT 500]
   RA643
   362.1969—dc23   2013025021

A catalog record for this book is available from the British Library.

*Special discounts are available for bulk purchases of this book. For more
information, please contact Special Sales at 410-516-6936 or specialsales@press
.jhu.edu.*

Johns Hopkins University Press uses environmentally friendly book
materials, including recycled text paper that is composed of at least 30
percent post-consumer waste, whenever possible.

Contents

Contributors

George Alleyne

Sir George Alleyne, a native of Barbados, became director of the Pan American Sanitary Bureau (PASB), Regional Office of the World Health Organization on February 1, 1995, and completed a second four-year term on January 31, 2003. In 2003 he was elected director emeritus of the PASB. From February 2003 until December 2010 he was the UN secretary general's special envoy for HIV/AIDS in the Caribbean. In October 2003 he was appointed chancellor of the University of the West Indies. He currently holds an adjunct professorship at the Bloomberg School of Public Health, Johns Hopkins University. Dr. Alleyne has received numerous awards in recognition of his work, including prestigious decorations and national honors from many countries in the Americas. In 1990, he was made knight bachelor by Queen Elizabeth II for his services to medicine. In 2001, he was awarded the Order of the Caribbean Community, the highest honor that can be conferred on a Caribbean national.

Louis Galambos

Louis Galambos is a professor of history at Johns Hopkins University and codirector of the Institute for Applied Economics, Global Health, and the Study of Business Enterprise. He has taught at Rice University, Rutgers University, and Yale University and has served as president of the Business History Conference and the Economic History Association. A former editor of the *Journal of Economic History*, Professor Galambos has written extensively on U.S. business history, on business-government relations, on the economic aspects of modern institutional development in America, and on the rise of the bureaucratic state. His central interest for some years has been the process of innovation in public, nonprofit, and private organizations. His most recent book is *The Creative Society—and the Price Americans Paid for It* (2012). Galambos also teaches a popular undergraduate course, "Global Public Health since World War II." One of the focal points of the course is the transition from support for healthcare systems in the developing world to support for disease-specific policies.

Stuart Gilmour

Stuart Gilmour has 15 years' experience of research in global health. He is currently an assistant professor in the Department of Global Health Policy at the University of Tokyo. Before coming to Japan, Mr. Gilmour was a research fellow in the UK's leading health policy think tank, the King's Fund. Originally from Australia, he worked as a statistician researching legal and illicit drug policy in Australia, where he helped to establish the Sydney Medically Supervised Injecting Centre. He has published on a diverse range of health topics, including the epidemiology of drug use, mental health, HIV and other infectious diseases, and health financing in developing nations.

Felicia Marie Knaul

Dr. Felicia Marie Knaul is an associate professor at Harvard Medical School and director of the Harvard Global Equity Initiative, where she serves as the codirector of the Secretariat for the Global Task Force on Expanded Access to Cancer Care and Control in Developing Countries, an initiative she helped to found in 2009 and for which she is lead author of the book *Closing the Cancer Divide*, released in 2012 by Harvard University Press. She is also a senior economist at the Mexican Health Foundation, where she has led a research group focused on health and the economy since 2000. After being diagnosed with breast cancer in 2007, she founded the Mexican nonprofit Tómatelo a Pecho to promote research and advocacy initiatives in Latin America. Dr. Knaul has held senior government posts in Mexico and Colombia and has worked for bilateral and multilateral agencies, including WHO, the World Bank, and UNICEF. She is a board member of numerous organizations, including the Union for International Cancer Control, and is author of more than 130 academic and policy publications.

Margaret E. Kruk

Dr. Margaret E. Kruk is an assistant professor of Health Policy and Management at Columbia University's Mailman School of Public Health. Dr. Kruk's research focuses on health system effectiveness and population preferences for healthcare in sub-Saharan Africa, including Tanzania, Ethiopia, Liberia, and Ghana. She has published on women's preferences for maternal healthcare, health systems effectiveness, healthcare financing, and evaluation of large-scale health programs in low-income countries. Previously, Dr. Kruk was an assistant professor in health management and policy at the University of Michigan School of Public Health and policy advisor for health at the Millennium Project, an advisory body to the UN Secretary General on the Millennium Development Goals.

Soeren Mattke

Dr. Soeren Mattke is a senior scientist at the RAND Corporation and the managing director of RAND Health Advisory Services, its consulting practice. Dr. Mattke is an expert in evaluating new technologies and products as well as innovative approaches to organizing and delivering health care services, especially for chronic care. He has worked with a long list of leading pharmaceutical, device, and health care technology companies and is helping clients worldwide regarding how to measure and communicate the value of their innovations. He is advising clients on strategic planning decisions, product approval applications, coverage and reimbursement strategy, post-market product development, and corporate communications. Previously, Dr. Mattke was the administrator, Health Policy Unit, Organisation for Economic Cooperation and Development.

Gustavo Nigenda

Dr. Gustavo Nigenda is a research associate at the Harvard Global Equity Initiative. Recently, he served as the director of Innovation Services and Health Systems and coordinator of the doctoral program on health systems at the Mexican National Institute of Public Health. He is also a member of the research group and a consultant for Cáncer de Mama: Tómatelo a Pecho, an initiative that aims to reduce breast cancer mortality in Latin America through early detection and effective treatment. Dr. Nigenda has published extensively on various topics, including human resources for health, health policy, social health protection, and health system reforms in Mexico. Dr. Nigenda earned his PhD in health policy from the London School of Economics and Political Science. Since 1980, he has worked with research groups in the field of public health.

Sania Nishtar

In early April 2013, Dr. Sania Nishtar was appointed Caretaker Federal Minister for Education and Training, Science and Technology and Information Technology, in the government of Pakistan. She is the founder and president of the NGO think tank Heartfile, which today is the most powerful health policy voice in Pakistan and is recognized as a model for replication in other developing countries. Her areas of interest are health systems, global health, broader issues of governance, and public-private relationships. In Pakistan, her pioneering work in the health sector has inspired new initiatives and shaped policies on health reform and noncommunicable diseases. She is also the founder of Pakistan's Health Policy Forum and provides support to many agencies in an advisory role. Dr. Nishtar is a member of many expert working groups and task forces of the World Health Organization and is currently a board member of both the International Union for Health Promotion and the Alliance for Health Policy and Systems Research. She is also a member of the World Economic Forum's Global Agenda Council, the Clinton Global Initiative, the Ministerial Leadership Initiative for Global Health, and many other international initiatives. Formerly, she was on several international boards and chaired several global campaigns and programs. She has also been an advisor to WHO on numerous occasions, has published over 100 journal articles, and is the author of 6 books.

Kenji Shibuya
Dr. Shibuya has been a key figure in supporting Japan's role in global health. He founded the Japan Institute for Global Health, which is working with a variety of sectors, including academia, government, industry, and the media, to promote global health in Japan. He also established the innovative Global Health Leadership Program at the University of Tokyo, where he is currently faculty chair. Previously, Dr. Shibuya was a research fellow at the Harvard Center for Population and Development Studies. He also worked in WHO's Global Program on Evidence for Health Policy and was a coordinator for the Health Statistics and Evidence Unit from 2005 until 2008. He has published extensively on mortality, causes of death, burden of disease, risk factors, cost effectiveness, priority setting, and health system performance assessment.

Lisa Smith
Lisa Smith is a research specialist with the William Davidson Institute Healthcare Research Initiative at the University of Michigan. Smith uses multidisciplinary research to generate new evidence and policy advice to inform improvements in global access to healthcare goods and services in developing countries. Her research is focused on innovative methods for improving the global market for healthcare commodities and public and private sector supply chains for such commodities within countries. She coordinates and manages research partnerships with a number of global development organizations.

Jeffrey L. Sturchio

Dr. Jeffrey L. Sturchio is a visiting scholar at the Institute for Applied Economics, Global Health, and the Study of Business Enterprise at Johns Hopkins University and senior partner at Rabin Martin, a leading global health strategy consulting firm. From 2009 to 2011, he was president and CEO of the Global Health Council, where he established the NCD Roundtable. Before joining the council, Dr. Sturchio was vice president, Corporate Responsibility, at Merck & Co., Inc., president of The Merck Company Foundation, and Chairman of the U.S. Corporate Council on Africa, whose 160 member companies represent some 85% of U.S. private sector investment in Africa. He was a member of the board of the African Comprehensive HIV/AIDS Partnerships in Botswana (2005–9) and a member of the private sector delegation to the Board of the Global Fund to Fight AIDS, TB and Malaria (2002–8). He is currently chairman of the BroadReach Institute for Training and Education and a member of the boards of the U.S. Pharmacopeia and the Museum of AIDS in Africa. Dr. Sturchio is also a senior associate of the Global Health Policy Center at the Center for Strategic and International Studies; a principal of the Modernizing Foreign Assistance Network; a fellow of the American Association for the Advancement of Science; and a member of the Council on Foreign Relations. He has published widely on global health, corporate responsibility, public-private partnerships, and the history of chemistry and the pharmaceutical industry and is a regular contributor to the *Huffington Post*. He received his AB in history from Princeton University and a PhD in the history and sociology of science from the University of Pennsylvania.

Brian White-Guay

Dr. Brian White-Guay trained as a physician and is currently a professor on the Faculty of Pharmacy of the Université de Montreal, where he is responsible for an undergraduate program in biopharmaceutical sciences and is also involved in research programs on drug utilization and prediction of response to treatments. Dr. White-Guay previously worked for over 20 years with Merck & Co. Inc. and held senior positions in the United States and Europe in clinical operations and global regulatory affairs. His professional interests include innovation in drug discovery and development, clinical trial design and evaluation, and the regulation of medicines in projects carried out in Europe, Canada, and the United States.

Prashant Yadav

Dr. Prashant Yadav is director of the Healthcare Research Initiative in the William Davidson Institute at the University of Michigan. He also holds faculty appointments at the Ross School of Business and the School of Public Health at the University of Michigan. A leading expert on pharmaceutical and healthcare supply chains in developing countries, Dr. Yadav's research explores the functioning of healthcare supply chains using a combination of empirical, analytical, and qualitative approaches. He is the author of many scientific publications, and his work has been featured in prominent print and broadcast media. He serves on the advisory boards of many public and private organizations in the field of global health.

Acknowledgments

We thank our fellow members of the NCD Working Group for their engagement and sound advice: Sir George Alleyne (former director, Pan American Health Organization; University of the West Indies; and Bloomberg School of Public Health, Johns Hopkins University), Robert Black (Bloomberg School of Public Health, Johns Hopkins University), Felicia Marie Knaul (Harvard Global Equity Initiative), Margaret E. Kruk (Mailman School of Public Health, Columbia University), Richard Laing (World Health Organization), Soeren Mattke (RAND Corporation), Sania Nishtar (Heartfile Pakistan), Tom Quinn (Center for Global Health, Johns Hopkins University), Kenji Shibuya (Tokyo University), Brian White-Guay (Université de Montreal), and Prashant Yadav (University of Michigan).

We thank Smita Baruah and Craig Moscetti, formerly with the Global Health Council, for their collaboration during the early phases of this project. At Johns Hopkins, project managers Uttam Bajwa and Rachel Whitehead have been indispensable, along with Tina Flores and Kathy Chase-Gaudreau at Rabin Martin. They provided much of the day-to-day support that made this project and publication possible. James Hospedales (then at PAHO), Mario Ottiglio (IFPMA), Alec van Gelder (Astra Zeneca) and Tonya Villafana (World Bank) supported the consultations of the NCD Working Group and offered important insights of their own along the way. We thank the speakers and audience at a seminar we organized in February 2012 at the Council on Foreign Relations in Washington, DC, for their critical reactions. Kelley Squazzo and her colleagues at Johns Hopkins University Press believed in this book. We also gratefully acknowledge the support of the International Federation of Pharmaceutical Manufacturers & Associations, which sponsored a grant to Johns Hopkins University. Sponsored Research at Hopkins handled the grant with its customary combination of care and efficiency.

Noncommunicable Diseases in the Developing World

Closing the Gap

Jeffrey L. Sturchio and Louis Galambos

Noncommunicable diseases (NCDs)—including cardiovascular disease, diabetes, asthma and chronic respiratory infections, and cancers—are the leading causes of death worldwide. An estimated 36 million people die from such diseases each year, or roughly two out of three deaths globally; 80% of these fatalities occur in low- and middle-income countries (LMICs). The statistics are stark, yet they hide the human toll of such disease burdens. Think of the attention and resources given to AIDS, tuberculosis, and malaria over the past 20 years—and the dramatic progress we've seen in the fight against these infectious diseases. Yet TB and malaria killed between 1 and 2 million people worldwide in 2010. Cancers killed 8 million people in 2010, a number one-third higher than in 1990. The picture is similar for other NCDs: one in four deaths globally from heart disease or stroke, 1.3 million deaths from diabetes. This is a global epidemic. At current rates, there will be a 17% increase in the NCD burden over the next decade. But this burden is not evenly distributed: Africa will see a growth of greater than 25%, and the absolute number of deaths will be greatest in the Western Pacific and Southeast Asia regions.[1]

Millions of these deaths are preventable, both through programs aimed at reducing high-risk behaviors (tobacco use, alcohol abuse, poor diet, lack of physical activity) and ameliorating high-risk environments and also through improved treatment and service delivery for patients who need chronic care. Cost-effective interventions to reduce the burden of these diseases exist now, and sustained action can prevent millions of premature deaths. The global health community has become increasingly aware of NCDs as primary threats to individuals, communities, health system infrastructures, and economic development. It is now acknowledged that NCDs contribute greatly to rising healthcare costs and the loss of economic productivity.

A range of programs and interventions has been considered and some innovative efforts are under way, but positive outcomes have often been difficult to secure because of global inequities in healthcare access, the globalization of risk factors—many of which originate outside the health sector—and the costs of implementing interventions. In low- and middle-income countries, where the disease burden is transitioning from communicable to noncommunicable diseases, many populations are currently suffering from a double burden. This conclusion was made clear in the results of the Global Burden of Disease Study 2010, published in the *Lancet* in December 2012.[2]

A global movement for action on NCDs has been gathering momentum in recent years. The United Nations General Assembly passed a resolution on the prevention and control of NCDs in 2010. The NCD Alliance, a coalition of civil society organizations now led by Cary Adams of the Union for International Cancer Control, was created that fall. A year later, in September 2011, the UN convened a High-level Meeting on the Prevention and Control of Non-communicable Diseases, leading to adoption of a political declaration that laid out a clear plan for global surveillance of, monitoring of, and health system response to the prevention and control of NCDs. In May 2012, the World Health Organization's 65th World Health Assembly (WHA) set the first voluntary global targets for a 25% reduction in premature mortality from NCDs by 2025. These targets were confirmed in January 2013 by the WHO Executive Board and were debated at the 66th World Health Assembly in May 2013.

There are clear roles for the private sector as well as the public sector and civil society to work together in addressing the challenges posed by the noncommunicable disease burden. Yet given the global fiscal crisis of recent years, it is unrealistic to expect large pools of new resources from traditional donors. Policy makers need to decide how best to incorporate NCD responses into existing funding streams and programs. We need recommendations for action that are sustainable in the current political and economic landscape.

This was the context in which the Johns Hopkins Institute for Applied Economics, Global Health, and the Study of Business Enterprise convened an NCD Working Group of leading scholars to analyze gaps in NCD research, policy, and practice to make actionable recommendations to close the gaps.[3] The working group built on the 2011 RAND Report "Improving Access to Medicines for Noncommunicable Diseases in the Developing World" and consulted with experts at the World Bank and the Pan American Health Organization, among others. They explored a wide range of issues that governments and their partners must address to make sustainable progress in building a strong response to the NCD challenge. These include large questions around regional and national variations in the burden of NCDs and associated risk factors, how best to incorporate strategies for reducing NCD risk factors into existing national and international public health initiatives, and how to find new resources to finance the scale-up of NCD interventions. Through those discussions, the NCD Working Group came to a consensus around several key areas for policy intervention that will help to catalyze progress in NCD prevention and treatment in lower- and middle-income countries. They focused on five areas where health systems need strengthening to address gaps in the provision of NCD care and treatment and where the private sector can bring its expertise to bear on the problems: (1) accelerating regulatory harmonization, (2) structuring supply chains, (3) improving access to interventions, (4) restructuring primary care, and (5) promoting multisectoral action.[4]

The chapters that follow review these issues and provide recommendations for action based on the authors' experiences and insights. This introduction provides a framework for understanding the salience of these policy questions. We begin with reflections on how the call to action on noncommunicable diseases emerged on the global health agenda in recent years, then outline the movement that led to the UN system's response, as detailed in the September 2011 High-level Meeting. We then turn to the path forward: what needs to be done to achieve effective and sustainable global action on NCDs?

Chronic Disease and a Call to Action

In the aftermath of World War II, relationships between the economically developed and the developing world took a major turn for the better. New international institutions, including the United Nations, the World Health Organization, the Pan American Health Organization, the World Bank, the International Monetary Fund, and an amazing array of nongovernmental organizations, had a central role in this global transition. The breakup of the colonial empires and the collapse of communism in Eastern Europe near the end of the century accelerated progress toward a new international order that sought to avoid another world war and to foster trade, economic growth, and better health in all of the nations, large and small.

The progress toward these goals, including improved health, was uneven. All of the new institutions were learning by doing, and that is never a linear process, a single-file march toward a better world. The mistakes and conflicts of the late twentieth century are well recorded and remembered, at times to the exclusion of progress. Yet even a casual examination of the figures on mortality and morbidity incisively indicates what has been accomplished in healthcare. While much remains to be done, the average figures on global life expectancy provide telling evidence that the new postwar order has been, on balance, successful in improving the health of humankind. According to the UN Population Division, global average life expectancy at birth (for both sexes) increased from about 48 years in 1950–55 to roughly 68 years in 2005–10.[5]

Innovations in the medical sciences played a central role in this transformation. Advances in the use of cell cultures and ensuing developments in vaccine production and distribution were extremely important in preventing infectious diseases in first the developed and then the developing worlds. While malaria, HIV/AIDS, and drug-resistant diseases continued to pose perplexing challenges to medical researchers, the new international organizations, their private-sector partners, and healthcare professionals around the world could not help but be pleased by the accomplishments they had logged. The great disease-specific, vertical campaigns (that is, those employing a series of linked institutions all focusing on a specific disease or diseases) to improve immunization rates around the world were astonishing successes that could not have been imagined before World War II.[6]

Since the adoption of the UN's Millennium Development Goals in 2000, the global health community has focused mainly on maternal and child health and on HIV/AIDS, TB, and malaria. In dealing with HIV infections, for instance, more than eight million patients in lower- and middle-income countries now have access to life-saving antiretroviral treatments.[7] In addition, substantial resources are being devoted to malaria prevention and treatment; so, too, is the case with drug-resistant TB, a subject that has recently been front-page news in the *Wall Street Journal*.[8]

As so often happens in life, however, progress relentlessly uncovers—and normally breeds—new problems. This is certainly the case in global health. Economic growth in the developing world was encouraging, but it brought to the fore many "lifestyle" diseases that have created a "dual burden" in many LMICs; in addition to their ongoing efforts to prevent and treat infectious diseases, they are now faced with increasing incidences of diabetes, cardiovascular disease (CVD), asthma, and cancers. The toll taken by noncommunicable diseases forced physicians, the international organizations, and governments to search for new ways to deal with what had become the leading causes of death worldwide. New resources were clearly needed. A 2010 study by Rachel Nugent and Andrea Feigl of the Center for Global Development found that in 2007, only 2.3% ($503.3 million) of nearly $22 billion in Official Development Assistance (ODA) for health (that is, bilateral and multilateral aid from the OECD donors) went to NCDs. It was not much better in 2008, when the total was just $686 million of $26.4 billion.[9] Another recent estimate shows that the World Health Organization spent just 6% of its budget on NCDs, at a time when 36 million of the 57 million global deaths (or 3 out of 5) were attributable to NCDs.

Two other recent studies help to show the magnitude of the problem. The World Economic Forum estimated in September 2011 that if we continue with the status quo, NCDs will cost LMICs around $500 billion each year between now and 2025, for a total of more than $7 trillion. Indeed, Margaret Chan, director general of the WHO, has called them the "diseases that break the bank." A companion study by the World Health Organization modeled a range of cost-effective, evidence-based individual and sociopolitical interventions (or "best buys")—such as taxes on tobacco and alcohol, smoke-free workplaces and public spaces, increased health promotion campaigns, reduced consumption of salt, sugar, and trans fats, increased physical activity, and enhanced screening and treatment for CVD, cervical cancer, and hepatitis B. Together, these interventions could save millions of lives each year at a cost of only $11.4 billion (that's less than 3% of the total annual economic costs of NCDs). But neither governments nor donors have made these actions priorities.[10]

Changing this situation so that global priorities are better aligned with the global burden of disease is like turning a giant oil tanker to follow a new course. It won't be done quickly or easily. It will require an international research agenda and political campaign of the sort we've seen beginning to develop over the past few years. This early phase of the global movement—involving UN member states, nongovernmental organizations (NGOs), public health professionals, and the private sector—has attempted to refocus attention on the NCD challenge.[11]

The challenge is great. As we've mentioned, NCDs account for more than three-fifths of all deaths globally. Four-fifths of these deaths occur in lower- and middle-income countries, and nearly 30% of NCD deaths are avoidable. This means, for instance, that some 8.35 million people in developing countries die unnecessarily each year due to NCDs. These diseases are the leading causes of death and disability worldwide and are both caused by and a cause of poverty. If current trends continue, the burden of chronic disease will grow to more than 75% of deaths by 2030. The World Economic Forum, in their annual Global Risk Report for 2010, named NCDs as the third most important risk facing the globe, greater than food price volatility, oil price spikes, fiscal crises, or infectious diseases.[12]

Many of the risk factors associated with NCDs are related to modifiable behaviors, such as tobacco use, unhealthy diets, physical inactivity and harmful use of alcohol. Indeed, the WHO estimates that some 80% of NCD deaths could be avoided if people changed risky behaviors into health-seeking behaviors (stopping smoking, exercising more regularly, eating healthier foods, etc.). In the developing world alone, that could lead to more than 6 million avoided deaths annually.[13]

Let's look at the four major categories of NCDs in more detail. Cardiovascular disease remains the leading cause of death worldwide, accounting for more than 17 million deaths (7.3 million from heart attacks and 6.2 million due to stroke). Cancers are the second leading cause of death, with more than 7.6 million people succumbing each year. Chronic respiratory diseases (including asthma and chronic obstructive pulmonary disease) collectively account for 4.2 million deaths per year, and diabetes results in about 1.3 million deaths. Death and disability from NCDs is not evenly distributed. Take cancer, for instance—more than 7 in 10 cancer deaths occur in developing countries, where lung cancer and liver cancer are the biggest killers of men, breast cancer and cervical cancer of women. For some cancers, there is an even more stark disparity in outcomes: 90% of children who contract leukemia in developed countries are cured, while 90% of children who contract leukemia in the poorest 25 countries die. Whatever the income level of countries, NCDs are among the top 10 causes of death worldwide. If current trends continue, Africa will see the largest percentage increase (close to 25%) in deaths from NCDs by 2015, while Southeast Asia and the Western Pacific will have the highest absolute number of deaths.[14]

Another way of understanding the burden of NCDs is to look at the impact these conditions are having on a country and regional level. In Brazil, for instance, more than 70% of all deaths were due to NCDs in 2007, and NCDs were also the main source of disease burden. The good news was that age-standardized mortality declined by 20% between 1996 and 2007, thanks to successful public health programs, but at the same time diabetes and hypertension rose in parallel with excess weight.[15]

South Africa is experiencing a health transition characterized by the emergence of noncommunicable diseases in both rural and urban areas in addition to existing burdens of infectious disease, perinatal and maternal conditions, and injury-related disorders. There are increasing numbers of deaths from diabetes, chronic kidney disease, and cancer of the prostate and cervix (though deaths attributable to stroke, chronic obstructive airways disease, and lung cancer have fallen in recent years). The need for chronic care for both communicable and noncommunicable diseases is placing extraordinary demands on the South African healthcare system and producing calls for new integrated models of care.[16]

In India, chronic diseases (including mental disorders) are the leading causes of death and disability, and their impact is expected to continue increasing during the next 25 years due to a rapidly aging population. Risk factors are very common throughout the Indian population. A wide range of cost-effective primary and secondary prevention strategies is available, but coverage is low.[17] In Southeast Asia more generally, NCDs cause three-fifths of all deaths. Their prevalence is due in large part to widespread tobacco use, unhealthy diets, and inadequate physical activity. These risk factors are increasing because of urbanization, lack of access to healthy food choices, and a public health system that lacks adequate resources and surveillance systems at the primary care level. As the authors of a review of the southeast Asia situation indicate, "Inaction affects millions of lives—and often . . . the lives of those who have the least."[18] Their conclusion applies with equal force to Brazil, South Africa, and India, where NCDs often have the greatest effect on the poor; in fact, the inequality in risk factors and disease impact between groups of lower socioeconomic status and those of higher socioeconomic status appears to be a global phenomenon.[19]

So, to summarize: by 2010, several things were clear. NCDs were a growing global problem that was getting worse. They affected a large fraction of the world's population, with disproportionate effects on the poor and those living in lower- and middle-income countries. The economic impact of NCDs would in coming decades be measured in the trillions, and we faced a tsunami of disease that would overwhelm health systems if nothing were done. Rather than responding to the alarms from advocates and experts, however, governments and multilateral organizations responded slowly if at all. Why?

One important reason is that several myths about NCDs were widely established: first, that it was *unnecessary* to do anything about them, since dealing with other diseases (e.g., AIDS, TB, malaria) was more urgent. Even if one could be persuaded that NCDs were a serious problem, the next myth was the belief that addressing them was an *unattainable* goal, given other priorities and the lack of additional resources. It was assumed that if priorities were reset and additional resources were found, NCD prevention and control would still be *unaffordable*. This attitude justified maintaining the status quo. Finally, even if not unaffordable and attainable, it was *inappropriate* to address them, given the need to stay focused on AIDS, TB and malaria, or maternal and child health.[20]

The UN System Responds: The High-level Meeting on Prevention and Control of Non-communicable Diseases

Fortunately, a number of interested groups advocated aggressive action against NCDs. The High-level Meeting (HLM) itself was an important forum for those who wanted to reorient the global health community. The impetus for the mid-2010 UN resolution setting up the HLM—only the second time the General Assembly devoted a special session to a health issue—came from the Caribbean Community (CARICOM) nations, which found themselves challenged by a growing prevalence of NCDs in the context of increasing pressure on resources. After placing the issue on the UN agenda, the Caribbean countries continued to advocate for other member states to join the cause. The movement began to grow.[21]

The range of response to the calls for action consisted of a complex mix of public health imperatives, practical realities, and political calculations. As Devi Sridhar, Peter Piot, and Steve Morrison observed in a paper for the Center for Strategic and International Studies, it would be important to "get the politics right." In their view (and drawing on the lessons of success following the 2001 HIV/AIDS UN General Assembly Special Session), this would entail: (1) focusing on the key diseases and risk factors, with adequate data to catalyze action; (2) providing motivated leadership, especially by the UN secretary general, the WHO director-general, and the NCD Alliance; (3) developing specific, feasible, measurable goals; and (4) blending those goals with national plans (including financing, regulation, cross-sectoral initiatives, and tobacco control). The NCD Alliance launched its civil society network in September 2010 at the Millennium Summit, and the race toward the NCD HLM was on.[22]

The High-level Meeting presented a crucial opportunity to place the issues around NCDs on the global agenda. This was a critical step in persuading countries to adopt feasible recommendations for action that would affect everyday practices in communities and clinics around the world. This political process, like all political processes, would be determined by competing interests and the relative power of the groups representing those interests. Thus, the result of the HLM—the Political Declaration on the Prevention and Control of Non-communicable Diseases adopted by the General Assembly on September 20—embodies a negotiated consensus of all of those competing factions. As is always true of an international compromise, hardly anyone was completely satisfied with the final Political Declaration. Nevertheless, it provides a sound basis for the work that must now be done to make progress in the fight against NCDs. As with most UN declarations, the commitments made by the member states are declarations of intent. They provide a framework for action and a catalyst to mobilize the necessary resources and coalitions of like-minded actors to effect change.[23]

Who were some of the key parties involved, and what were their interests? The formal players at the UN were the member states themselves, from both developed and developing countries. The latter, including most of the CARICOM countries, who had started the ball rolling, are concerned about the social and economic impact NCDs are having on their populations and the relative lack of resources to pay for the necessary programs to address them. The donor countries—including the United States, Canada, the European Union, and Japan—shared that concern but were wary of adopting new financial obligations to pay for the programs required in developing countries at a time of financial crisis in most of their economies. As these countries recognized, NCDs were just one of a number of competing international policy priorities, including the Millennium Development Goals (MDGs), poverty reduction, climate change, food security, and the perennial favorites security, economic development, and UN reform.

On all these issues sharp divisions existed within the UN member states themselves. The G77, for instance, took a view sharply at odds with the major donors (such as the United States and the EU), focusing on the need to change trade rules to enable LMICs to gain improved access to the essential medicines required to treat NCDs. They invoked the use of the Agreement on Trade Related Aspects of Intellectual Property Rights flexibilities to get around patents as barriers to access. In an effort to achieve a consensus, the WHO had coordinated a process of consultation and negotiation among the member states and other concerned stakeholders. These included the WHO itself and other intergovernmental organizations (UNICEF, the UN Population Fund, the World Bank, the World Trade Organization, etc.).

On display was civil society in all its complexity, including academic researchers from universities like Johns Hopkins, public health professionals, NGOs (eventually represented by the NCD Alliance), faith-based organizations, the private sector, and the media. All had a role to play in the dialogue that led to the HLM and also the conversation at the HLM itself, which was a three-ring circus of people and organizations looking for a way for their voices to be heard and their views incorporated in the Political Declaration that was likely to emerge from the UN. That explains, in part, why during the General Assembly week in mid-September, there were more than 100 side events at hotels and other meeting venues around Manhattan. In these gatherings, each of the groups held forth on why their priority—sports, agriculture, women and girls, diet and nutrition, to name just a few—was critical to achieving the outcomes required for effectively meeting the challenge of NCDs.

Three of these groups were particularly influential: proponents of primary care; NGOs; and the private sector. Advocates of primary care used the HLM meeting as an opportunity to make their case, noting that "integrated primary care is essential for tackling NCDs" and that "better outcomes occur by addressing diseases through an integrated approach in a strong primary care system." This approach, they argued, would advance the effort to "address complexity in health problems, in both developed and developing countries," by putting "people and their values at the centre of the process." The answer was to invest more in people-centered primary care. To the $9 billion per year needed to pay for the right interventions, they would add an additional $9 billion to strengthen primary care services and ensure a supply of well-trained health professionals.[24] This proposal ran counter to the thoughts of the countries that did not want to take on any additional financial commitments, a point to which we'll return.

NGOs were represented in large part by the NCD Alliance, a broad coalition led by the International Diabetes Federation, the World Heart Federation, the Union for International Cancer Control and the International Union Against Tuberculosis and Lung Disease and a number of Summit Partners, including the American Cancer Society and the Global Health Council (of which Jeffrey Sturchio was then the CEO). The NCD Alliance, which represented more than 2,000 grassroots organizations, provided a strong voice for the interests of patients and families living with noncommunicable diseases. If governments "continue to ignore the threat of NCDs," the organizations argued, "we will sleepwalk into a future in which healthy people will be in a minority, obese and unhealthy children die before their parents, and economic development and already vulnerable health systems are overwhelmed." They called in particular for national plans to deal with NCDs, for time-based targets, for new resources, and for clear accountability mechanisms to track progress against the commitments countries would make at the HLM.[25]

The private sector, for its part, also had an interest in tackling NCDs. Clearly, companies were in a position to bring important skills and resources to the tasks ahead. Pharmaceutical firms provide the necessary treatments for CVD, diabetes, asthma, and cancers; they continue to do a significant part of the research that produces better tools. Diagnostic and medical device companies also had a direct and obvious role to play. Food and beverage companies came into play by adopting voluntary standards to decrease the salt, sugar, and trans fats in their products to help counter the trend toward obesity and its associated NCDs. Companies in other sectors (including sports and entertainment) also offered proposals and expressed their interest in working with other stakeholders to fight NCDs.

As anyone with experience in public health could have anticipated, the private sector's involvement stirred up some intense controversy. Everyone agreed that the firms in the tobacco industry were pariahs, since tobacco use was one of the key factors leading to millions of deaths each year from lung diseases and cancers. Seeking a more extended front and decisive action, a group of 140 NGOs formed the Alliance Against Conflict of Interest and raised a concern about any UN engagement with "private sector and trade associations whose products and marketing contribute to the development of NCDs." They argued for a regulatory approach to industry, rather than the collaborative approach based on voluntary standards and favored by most industries. One advocate likened the latter to "letting Dracula advise on blood-bank security."[26]

As you can imagine, the negotiations around the Political Declaration of the HLM were full of drama, ideological commitments, and straightforward interest struggles. What was the outcome of this year of collecting and sifting evidence, of policy papers and consultations, and of seemingly endless meetings and discussions around the world? Central to the results was the UN acknowledgment that the global burden and threat of NCDs "constitutes one of the major challenges for development in the 21st century" and threatens the achievement of the MDGs. The UN noted "with profound concern" that NCDs represented a challenge of "epidemic proportions," affecting everyone. The Declaration pointed to a range of linked effects and causes—poverty, obesity, gender issues, maternal and child health, HIV/AIDS—and the need for integrated responses and health system strengthening.

The UN Political Declaration also pointed out that tackling the NCDs effectively requires "whole of government" and "whole of society" solutions. National policies and health systems would need to be strengthened. Various specific risk factors should be addressed and policy makers would need to focus on creating health-promoting environments. All stakeholders need to be involved, the UN noted, not just governments. Efforts need to be internationally coordinated, working across borders and through collaborative, multi-stakeholder partnerships (including civil society and the private sector, "where appropriate"). Research and development had an important role to play, and monitoring and evaluation must be part of the effort if we were going to know what worked and why. Additional resources would be required.

In addition to these policy prescriptions, the UN General Assembly called for four major deliverables: by 2012, the WHO would issue a global monitoring framework, including indicators and voluntary targets for governments to consider; also by 2012, the WHO would issue a new framework for multisectoral partnerships that could be incorporated into national policies;[27] by 2013, the secretary general would report back to the UN General Assembly on progress; and by 2014, there would be a comprehensive progress report on the implementation of the Political Declaration at the national and global levels.

What was not stated in the Political Declaration was almost as interesting as what was included. One observer noted in *Lancet Oncology* that this was "more a politically correct declaration than a political declaration of war." It avoided hard targets. There was no accountability mechanism. No significant new money was committed or pledged. There was no commitment to change existing trade rules and practices.[28] Others pointed to important lacunae in the disease conditions taken up by the General Assembly. Where were mental, neurological, and substance abuse disorders, which together account for nearly one-quarter of all years lived with a disability around the world and often occur together with other noncommunicable diseases, yet are not fully integrated into primary care settings, especially in lower- and middle-income countries?[29] What about the "long tail" of endemic NCDs—such as rheumatic heart disease—that affect as many as one billion people (many living in absolute poverty), that are not largely linked to the major lifestyle risk factors of the other NCDs, and that require responses focused on broader health system investments?[30] While these criticisms were certainly true, they were, from our perspective, less significant than the fact that the UN member states were unanimously on record about the importance of fighting the growing impact of NCDs.

The Path Forward: Toward Effective Global Action on NCDs

However, substantial ambiguity existed regarding the collective path forward. Almost as soon as the Political Declaration was announced, there was contention and foot-dragging among the WHO's member states about the global monitoring framework. The WHO responded with a global consultative process, with regional meetings to elicit input and guidance for the targets and indicators. But the debates at the January 2012 Executive Board meeting and at the May 2012 World Health Assembly in Geneva were intense and inconclusive, resulting in the deadline for a global monitoring framework being pushed back to 2013. The one clear outcome from the World Health Assembly was an agreement around a commitment to lower unnecessary deaths from NCDs by 25% by 2025 ("25 × 25").[31]

This agreement was seized on by advocates and champions of the NCD cause as the first bold target for a new global campaign against heart disease, cancers, diabetes, and chronic respiratory diseases, one that for the first time extended beyond the MDG goals in 2015. The fine print matters, of course, and the 25 × 25 target included less than meets the eye in terms of resources, specific roles, and responsibilities. Still, it was a dramatic start, and work continued on a number of fronts. The WHO doggedly pursued the official intergovernmental process, while the NCD Alliance and other advocates continued to call for more ambitious outcomes. The result, in November 2012, was agreement on a preliminary set of targets and indicators that were debated by the WHO Executive Board and then placed before the World Health Assembly in May 2013. These emerged from a formal meeting that included representatives of 119 member states, one regional economic integration organization, one intergovernmental organization, and 17 NGOs. This diverse group was able to agree on 25 indicators to monitor trends in implementation, along with 9 voluntary global targets "for consideration by Member States"[32] (see figs. I.1 and I.2).

The targets are interesting. The participants reaffirmed the target of 25 × 25, noting that it would measure the relative reduction in overall mortality from the

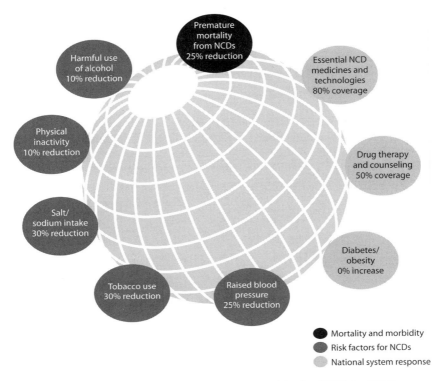

Fig. I.1. Nine voluntary global NCD targets proposed by the WHO for 2025. Courtesy of the World Health Organization.

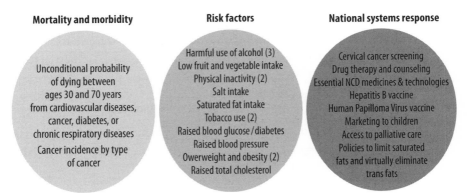

Fig. I.2. Indicators for NCD global monitoring framework proposed by the WHO. Total number of related indicators are in parentheses. Courtesy of the World Health Organization.

four NCDs for people between the ages of thirty and seventy. Most of the other targets dealt with risk factors, rather than specific diseases, and only two dealt with the general health system response:

- at least a 10% relative reduction in the harmful use of alcohol, as appropriate, within the national context
- a 10% relative reduction in the prevalence of insufficient physical activity
- a 30% relative reduction in mean population intake of salt/sodium
- a 30% relative reduction in prevalence of current tobacco use in persons aged 15+ years
- a 25% relative reduction in the prevalence of raised blood pressure or contain the prevalence of raised blood pressure according to national circumstances
- halt the rise in diabetes and obesity
- at least 50% of eligible people receive drug therapy and counseling (including glycaemic control) to prevent heart attacks and strokes
- an 80% availability of the affordable basic technologies and essential medicines, including generics, required to treat major noncommunicable diseases in both public and private facilities[33]

This step forward followed the normal pattern for voluntary public health programs. The monitoring framework immediately provoked a chorus of outcries over what was left out. Why, it was asked, was there not more on specific disease targets? Why wasn't there more of an effort to provide a specific roadmap for how to achieve these targets? Where were the explicit links between the health agenda and the post-2015 development agenda? The complaints poured forth from all sides. But the debate was now on the ground the WHO had staked out for this innovation in global public health. A partial consensus had been achieved on a series of steps, measures that could never encompass everything that every nation, every international organization, and every NGO wanted. The next step was to frame the WHO's action plan for implementing these recommendations by 2020 and to improve the focus on outcomes, which—along with the targets and indicators of the Global Monitoring Framework and a proposed Global Coordinating Mechanism—was to be debated at the 66th World Health Assembly in May 2013.[34] At the same time, attention is beginning to turn to the evolving discussion on post-2015 sustainable development goals, so the outcomes of the WHA debate will inevitably be cast in the broader context of how health will feature in the framework now being developed to build on the Millennium Development Goals. An emerging consensus states that health remains a key challenge to sustainable development and that NCDs, as crucial determinants of health, should be included in the new development agenda. But exactly how remains to be seen, as the global health system grapples with new governance challenges.[35]

The path forward on NCDs is and will always be contested. The debates and critiques will continue to pour out while healthcare workers continue to implement and refine a set of ambitious, measurable, time-bound, achievable targets and metrics on NCDs. The global monitoring framework will provide accountability if governments and their partners implement and support independent mechanisms to track progress and build capacity for coordinated, multisectoral actions at country, regional, and global levels to fulfill commitments made in the 2011 Political Declaration.[36] Those actions should develop along four related lines. First, there will be efforts to achieve better *integration* of NCDs with other health system priorities—whether HIV/AIDS, maternal or child health, or plans to improve the organization of clinics and hospitals at the national level. Second, this will be accompanied by new efforts for *implementation* of "best buys," the proven, cost-effective interventions that can help to prevent NCDs or to treat those that are most prevalent. Third, both integration and implementation will require attention to *innovation*: in new prevention strategies; new treatment modalities (e.g., combination treatments, or polypills, to address comorbidities such as hypertension, elevated cholesterol, and diabetes); and new multisectoral partnerships to address NCDs where people live, work, and play. Fourth, as always in healthcare, there will be a relentless search for additional *investment*, so that adequate resources are available to meet the NCD challenges.

As this newest phase in the global health movement gets under way, it is encouraging to look at a notable example of how to move forward. An article in the *Lancet* by Deborah Dowell and Thomas Farley of the New York City Department of Health and Mental Hygiene recounted a decade worth of efforts in New York City to use both voluntary and regulatory methods to "solve the problems with the largest effects" on the health of New Yorkers. These measures included:

- 2002: tobacco control campaign to protect New Yorkers from secondary smoke and to make smoking less convenient and easier to quit.
- 2002: increased taxes on cigarettes (which now cost $11 per pack)

- 2002: Smoke-Free Air Act (extended from restaurants and bars to public parks and beaches in 2011)
- 2006: NYC Board of Health restrictions on trans fats in restaurants
- 2006: restaurants required to post calorie counts on menus
- 2006–9: NYC Department of Transportation added 200 miles of bicycle lanes
- 2009: mandated bike parking inside office buildings
- 2009: NYC campaign stressing the health impact of sugar-sweetened beverages
- 2012: NYC Board of Health regulation limiting restaurant portion of sugar-sweetened beverages to 16 ounces[37]
- 2012: health-based standards for the 260 million meals and snacks purchased by city agencies (fruits and vegetables, calorie restrictions on beverages)
- 2012: participation in the National Salt Reduction Initiative (−25% in 5 years, in collaboration with food companies)[38]

What were the measurable results? New Yorkers' "life expectancy has remained higher and increased faster than that of Americans overall." There were remarkable changes in key indicators associated with improved health outcomes: a 35% reduction in smoking prevalence between 2002 and 2010; major decreases in daily consumption of sugar-sweetened beverages among adults; and doubling of commuter bicycling between 2006 and 2010.[39] New York's experience shows that changes in the social and physical environment mean that people are more likely to make healthy choices. It provides as well another argument for an intersectoral approach that looks not just at what health officials can do, but also what other stakeholders can contribute. Prevention of NCDs is not necessarily costly. Many health-promoting policies can be relatively inexpensive, and taxes on cigarettes, for instance, can be used to pay for NCD prevention.

Perhaps the most important lesson from New York City's experience is that high-level political commitment is essential. Mayor Michael R. Bloomberg has been a visible and persistent advocate for public health. In his speech to the HLM in September 2011, he noted that "while government action is not sufficient alone, it is nevertheless absolutely essential. There are powers only governments can exercise, policies only governments can mandate and enforce, and results only governments can achieve. To halt the worldwide epidemic of noncommunicable diseases, governments at all levels must make healthy solutions the default social option. That is, ultimately, government's highest duty."[40]

We all know that New York is a long way from Nairobi. But the factors that lead to success in meeting the challenge of NCDs apply equally in both developing and developed country environments. NCDs are now on the political agenda, which offers the opportunity for progress. As Mayor Bloomberg observed, government action is essential, if not sufficient, for success. We'll also need to see unified, inclusive, and focused civil society movements at the local, regional, country, and global levels. While the NCD Alliance has made important strides in this direction, much remains to be done.

Structure of the Book

In the spirit of intersectoral action, we offer the following five essays, each staking out a particular area of activity and concluding with specific steps that can be taken now to move ahead in the global campaign against NCDs.

Brian White-Guay reviews current challenges and future prospects for the global regulatory framework. Considerable work has been done on regulatory harmonization for medicines in recent years, but the whole has yet to add up to more than the sum of the parts. White-Guay recommends developing a common end-stage vision for regulatory convergence and then defining the most urgent priorities to improve access to essential medicines for treatment of NCDs and adopting clear indicators of results to measure progress. Opportunities include training and capacity-building efforts for national medicines regulatory authorities; exploration of regional harmonization programs (to apply new administrative procedures that can reduce inefficiency and waste); and the establishment of a network of quality control laboratories to limit the circulation of substandard or counterfeit medicines. Finally, more widespread deployment of IT solutions can facilitate communication and knowledge transfer among national medical regulatory authorities and stringent regulatory authorities in such areas as manufacturing licenses, import authorizations and certification of good manufacturing practices (GMPs).

Lisa Smith and Prashant Yadav conclude that to improve access to NCD medicines, we need to understand the structural obstacles in medicine supply chains and to rethink access from the level of the manufacturer to the level of the patient. This will require detailed study of global and national supply chains to address fragmentation of supply, which leads to poor economies of scale, poor coverage, and challenges in tracing products. Other potential solutions include establishing accredited healthcare retail networks to ensure availability of quality medicines at affordable prices and to encourage appropriate use, as well as wider use, of differential pricing. Smith and Yadav suggest testing these ideas in a targeted way, with initiatives in selected resource-limited settings that address diseases that cause the highest burden.

In his essay, Soeren Mattke addresses lessons learned from the response to the HIV epidemic in assessing how to improve the use of NCD interventions. He focuses on the importance of public-private partnerships for leveraging industry capabilities in support of improved NCD prevention, treatment, and care at the local level. Pharmaceutical and other healthcare companies can help improve both care delivery systems and research on ways to increase adherence to treatment (which will enhance long-term patient outcomes), in addition to the development of sustainable business models to upgrade access to medicines. Specific solutions include helping LMICs to develop context-appropriate treatment guidelines, training materials for healthcare providers, and patient education tools. Industry can also deploy its R&D expertise in the search for new medicines (such as polypills) to provide better solutions for NCD treatment in resource-limited settings, as well as experimenting with community-based approaches to improve care and treatment outcomes.

In their chapter, Margaret E. Kruk, together with Gustavo Nigenda and Felicia Marie Knaul, proposes an agenda for reconfiguring primary care to deal more effectively with the NCD challenge. They argue that "much of the opportunity in reducing the health and economic impacts of NCDs lies in prevention, early diagnosis, and treatment—the domain of primary care" and that primary care "is perfectly positioned to be the main platform for the health system response to NCDs." However, health systems in many lower- and middle-income countries are unprepared to tackle NCDs because of an existing focus on infectious disease and maternal and child health and constrained financial resources that make it difficult to take on new tasks. But by focusing on four key elements essential to the effective functioning of primary care in the NCD era—integration of care, innovations in service delivery, inclusion of communities and the voice of the patient, and making creative use of new information and communications technologies—health systems can provide high-quality, accessible care that responds to today's needs and builds the basis for resilience in taking on future challenges.

George Alleyne and Sania Nishtar begin by pointing out that the September 2011 Political Declaration "emphasized the critical need for a multisectoral response," mentioning it no less than 15 times. Their essay proposes a taxonomy of multisectoral action (among various government agencies outside of health, including education, energy, agriculture, sports, transport, communications, urban planning, environment, labor, employment, industry and trade, finance, and social and economic development) and intersectoral cooperation (working with the "whole of society," including the private sector and other nongovernmental organizations). Alleyne and Nishtar provide a careful analysis of the nature and possibilities of these different modes of sectoral cooperation and examine their relevance for translating the mandates of the Political Declaration into practical actions that will improve public health outcomes with respect to NCDs.

In the final chapter, Stuart Gilmour and Kenji Shibuya delineate several cross-cutting themes from the preceding essays and consider the implications for the NCD response of enhancing global health governance through improved coordination and collaboration and the engagement of nontraditional sectors in public health practice. They are optimistic that policy innovation in NCDs along the lines proposed in this volume offers "an opportunity to improve the equity, efficiency, and responsiveness of health systems for the betterment of all of society."

The focus throughout the essays is primarily on lower- and middle-income countries. Most of the specific measures recommended are intended for the private sector or public-private partnerships to implement. Together they comprise a pragmatic agenda for reducing the burden of NCDs and provide an initial roadmap for policy development and progress in the fight against these chronic conditions. All require the kind of leadership that Mayor Bloomberg has provided in his city and that the global health movement has seen in past decades in its highly successful campaigns against infectious diseases. We look forward to the lively debates and creative solutions that we hope these proposals will inspire.

NOTES

1. World Health Organization, Global status report on noncommunicable diseases, *2010*. Geneva: WHO, 2011.

2. See Horton R. GBD 2010: understanding disease, injury and risk. *Lancet* 380 (December 15/22/29, 2012): 2053–2054; Murray CLJ et al. GBD 2010: design, definitions and metrics. Ibid., 2063–2066; and the detailed papers in this *Lancet* special issue.

3. The members of the NCD Working Group are Sir George Alleyne (former director, Pan American Health Organization), Robert Black (Bloomberg School of

Public Health, Johns Hopkins University), Felicia Marie Knaul (Harvard Global Equity Initiative), Margaret E. Kruk (Mailman School of Public Health, Columbia University), Louis Galambos (Johns Hopkins University), Richard Laing (WHO), Soeren Mattke (RAND Corporation), Sania Nishtar (Heartfile Pakistan), Tom Quinn (Center for Global Health, Johns Hopkins University), Kenji Shibuya (Tokyo University), Jeffrey L. Sturchio (Rabin Martin and Johns Hopkins University), Brian White-Guay (Université de Montreal), and Prashant Yadav (University of Michigan).

4. These are clearly not the only policy questions raised by NCDs, but the members of the Working Group did feel that they represented priority cross-cutting themes that, if addressed effectively, would have an important impact on strengthening the global response.

There is of course a large and growing literature on the myriad aspects of research, policy and practice in NCDs: for complementary perspectives, see also Samb B, Desain N, Nishtar S, et al. Prevention and management of chronic disease: a litmus test for health-systems strengthening in low-income and middle-income countries. *Lancet* 376 (2010): 1785–1797; Rabkin M and El-Sadr WM. Why reinvent the wheel? Leveraging the lessons of HIV scale-up to confront non-communicable diseases. *Global Public Health* 6 (2011): 247–256; Narayan KMV, Ali MK, del Rio C, et al. Global noncommunicable diseases—lessons from the HIV/AIDS experience. *New England Journal of Medicine* 365 (2011): 876–878; Lamptey P, Merson M, Piot P, et al. Informing the 2011 UN session on non-communicable diseases: applying lessons from the AIDS response. *PLoS Medicine* 8 (2011): e1001086; Meiro-Lorenzo M, Villafana TL, and Harrit MN. Effective responses to non-communicable diseases: embracing action beyond the health sector. Health Nutrition and Population Sector Discussion Paper (Washington, DC: World Bank, 2011), www-wds.worldbank.org/external/default/WDS ContentServer/WDSP/IB/2011/11/03/000333037_20111103003702/Rendered /PDF/651320WP0Box360ctiveResponsestoNCDs.pdf; Nikolic I, Stanciole A, and Zaydman M. Chronic Emergency: Why NCDs Matter. Health, Nutrition, and Population Discussion Paper (Washington, DC: World Bank, 2011), http://siteresources .worldbank.org/HEALTHNUTRITIONANDPOPULATION/Resources/281627 -1095698140167/ChronicEmergencyWhyNCDsMatter.pdf; World Bank, Human Development Network. The growing emergency of non-communicable diseases: acting now to reverse course. Conference edition (Washington, DC: World Bank, September 2011), www-wds.worldbank.org/external/default/WDSContentServer/WDSP/IB/2011 /11/30/000386194_20111130023857/Rendered/PDF/657850WP0Box360C00WB DeepeningCrisis.pdf; Ebrahim S, Pearce N, Smeeth L, et al. Tackling non-communicable diseases in low- and middle-income countries: is the evidence from high-income countries all we need? *PLoS Medicine* 10 (January 2013): e1001377; Atun R, Jaffar S, Nishtar S, et al. Improving responsiveness of health systems to non-communicable diseases. *Lancet* 381 (February 23, 2013): 690–697; and Ali MK, Rabadan-Diehl C, Flanigan J, et al. Systems and capacity to address noncommunicable diseases in low- and middle-income countries. *Science Translational Medicine* 5 (April 17, 2013): 181cm4; and Lachat C, Otchere S, Roberfroid D, et al. Diet and physical activity for the prevention of noncommunicable diseases in low- and middle-income countries: a systematic policy review. *PLoS Medicine* 10 (June 2013): e1001465.

For useful multidisciplinary perspectives on addressing the challenge of NCDs, see the September 2011 special issue of the *Journal of Health Communications* developed by the World Economic Forum's Global Agenda Council on Chronic Disease and Wellness, edited by Anderson P and Nishtar S. Introduction: communicating the noncommunicable. *Journal of Health Communication* 16, supplement 2 (September 2011): 6–12. See also Stuckler D and Siegel K, eds., Sick Societies: Responding to the Global Challenge of Chronic Disease (Oxford: Oxford University Press, 2011), which synthesizes the evidence based on the prevention and control of NCDs from the perspectives of epidemiology, economics, health policy and management, and political economy, including how power and politics have impeded an effective global response to the challenge.

5. United Nations Population Division, Department of Economic and Social Affairs, World Population Prospects: The 2010 Revision, CD-ROM Edition. New York: UN, 2011, File 5-1: Life expectancy at birth (both sexes combined) by major area, region and country, 1950–2100 (years), Estimates, 1950–2010, POP/DB/WPP/Rev.2010/01/F05-1, http://esa.un.org/unpd/wpp/Excel-Data/mortality.html. Of course, this global average masks significant regional differences. In more developed regions of the world, life expectancy grew from about 66 years to roughly 77 years between 1950 and 2010, while in less developed regions—although the growth on average was more dramatic (from 42 years to about 66 years)—life expectancy in 2010 had only reached the level seen in developed countries half a century earlier. See also World Health Organization, Global Health Observatory. Mortality and Global Burden of Disease (GBD). WHO 2013, www.who.int/gho/mortality_burden_disease/en/index.html.

6. For an introduction to these historic immunization campaigns, see, for example, Gonzalez CL, Mass Campaigns and General Health Services (Geneva, World Health Organization, 1965), 7–59; Chumakov MP et al. Some Results of the Work on Mass Immunization in the Soviet Union with Live Poliovirus Vaccine Prepared from Sabin Strains. *Bulletin of the World Health Organization* 25 (1961): 79–91.

7. World Health Organization. 10 facts on HIV/AIDS. November 2012. www.who.int/features/factfiles/hiv/en/index.html.

8. See, for example, Otten M, Aregawi M, Were W, Karema C, Medin A, Bekele W, Jima D, et al. Initial evidence of reduction of malaria cases and deaths in Rwanda and Ethiopia due to rapid scale-up of malaria prevention and treatment. *Malaria Journal* 8, no. 1 (2009): 14; Anand G and McKay B. How Fight to Tame TB Made It Stronger. *Wall Street Journal*, (November 23, 2012): A1; Anand G and McKay B. Five Developing Nations Join to Fight Drug-Resistant TB. *Wall Street Journal*, (February 4, 2013): A9.

9. Chan KY, Adeloye D, Grant L, Kolčić I, and Marušić A. How big is the "next big thing"? Estimating the burden of non–communicable diseases in low- and middle-income countries. *Journal of Global Health* 2, no. 2 (December 2012): 020101;

Miszkurka M, Haddad S, Langlois ÉV, Freeman EE, Kouanda S, and Zunzunegui MV. Heavy burden of non-communicable diseases at early age and gender disparities in an adult population of Burkina Faso: World Health Survey. *BMC Public Health* 12, no. 1 (2012): 24; Nugent R and Feigl A. Where have all the donors gone? Scarce donor funding for non-communicable diseases. Center for Global Development, Working Paper 228, November 2010.

10. Bloom DE, Cafiero ET, Jané-Llopis E, et al. The Global Economic Burden of Noncommunicable Diseases. Geneva: World Economic Forum, 2011; Dr. Margaret Chan's Address at the High-level Meeting on Noncommunicable Diseases. United Nations General Assembly, New York, United States of America, 19 September 2011; World Health Organization. Scaling Up Action against Noncommunicable Diseases: How Much Will It Cost? Geneva: WHO, 2011.

11. Alwan AD, Galeab G, and Stuckler D. Development at risk: addressing non-communicable diseases at the United Nations high-level meeting. *Bulletin of the World Health Organization* issue 89 (2011): 546–546A; Beaglehole R, Bonita R, et al. UN High-Level Meeting on Non-Communicable Diseases: addressing four questions. *Lancet* 378 (July 30, 2011): 449–455; Coombes R. World leaders sign up to tackle causes of non-communicable diseases. *BMJ* 343 (September 21, 2011): d6034.

12. World Health Organization. Noncommunicable Diseases Country Profiles 2011; NCD Alliance. Tobacco: a major risk factor for Non-communicable Diseases. 2012; World Economic Forum. Global Risks 2010: A Global Risk Network Report. January 2010.

13. World Health Organization. Global Status Report on Noncommunicable Diseases 2010.

14. Global Health Observatory: NCD mortality and morbidity. World Health Organization, 2013, www.who.int/gho/ncd/mortality_morbidity/en/; Mackay J and Mensah G. The Atlas of Heart Disease and Stroke. World Health Organization, U.S. Centers for Disease Control, 2004; U.S. Institute of Medicine, Promoting Cardiovascular Health in the Developing World: A Critical Challenge to Achieve Global Health. Washington, DC: National Academies Press, 2010; Global Task Force on Expanded Access to Cancer Care and Control in Developing Countries, Report: Closing the Cancer Divide: A Blueprint to Expand Access in Low and Middle Income Countries, 2011; Knaul FM, Gralow JR, et al., eds., Closing the Cancer Divide: An Equity Imperative. Boston: Harvard Global Equity Initiative, 2012. See also Farmer P, Frenk J, Knaul FM, et al. Expansion of cancer care and control in countries of low and middle income: a call to action. *Lancet* 376 (October 2, 2010): 1186–1193; Smith SC, Collins A, Ferrari R, et al. Our time: a call to save preventable death from cardiovascular disease (heart disease and stroke). *Journal of the American College of Cardiology* 60 (December 4, 2012): 2343–2348.

15. Schmidt MI, Duncan BB, Azevedo e Silva G, et al. Chronic non-communicable diseases in Brazil: burden and current challenges. *Lancet* 377 (June 4, 2011): 1949–1961.

16. Mayosi BM, Flisher AJ, Lalloo UG, et al. The burden of non-communicable diseases in South Africa. *Lancet* 374 (September 12, 2009): 934–947.

17. Patel V, Chatterji S, Chisholm D, et al. Chronic diseases and injuries in India. *Lancet* 377 (January 29, 2011): 413–428.

18. Dans A, Ng N, Vargheses C, et al. The rise of chronic non-communicable diseases in southeast Asia: time for action. *Lancet* 377 (February 19, 2011): 680–689.

19. De Cesare M, Khang YH, Asaria P, et al. Inequalities in non-communicable diseases and effective responses. *Lancet* 381 (February 16, 2013): 585–597.

20. Here we follow the formulation of the myths surrounding NCDs articulated by Felicia Knaul and K. Srinath Reddy in a plenary session on the subject at the 2011 annual conference of the Global Health Council in Washington, DC. This is developed further for the case of cancer in Knaul FM, Gralow JR, Atun R, and Bhadelia A, eds. Closing the Cancer Divide: An Equity Imperative (Boston: Harvard Global Equity Initiative, 2012), 4–8. See also Knaul FM, Atun R, Farmer P, and Frenk J. Seizing the opportunity to close the cancer divide. *Lancet* 381 (June 29, 2013): 2238–2239.

21. Alleyne G, Stuckler D, and Alwan A. The hope and the promise of the UN Resolution on non-communicable diseases. *Globalization and Health* 6 (2010): 15; Samuels TA, Guell C, Legetic B, and Unwin N. Policy initiatives, culture and the prevention and control of chronic non-communicable diseases (NCDs) in the Caribbean. *Ethnicity & Health* ahead-of-print (2012): 1–19; T. A. Samuels TA and Hospedales CJ. From Port-of-Spain Summit to United Nations High Level Meeting: CARICOM and the global non-communicable disease agenda. *West Indian Medical Journal* 60, no. 4 (2011): 387–391.

22. Sridhar D, Morrison JS, and Piot P. Getting the politics right for the September 2011 UN High-Level Meeting on Non-Communicable Diseases. Center for Strategic and International Studies Global Health Policy Center, February 2011. http://csis.org/files/publication/110215_Sridhar_GettingPoliticsRight_Web.pdf.

23. United Nations General Assembly. Political Declaration of the High-level Meeting of the General Assembly on the Prevention and Control of Non-communicable Diseases, document A/66/L.1. 16 September 2011, www.un.org/ga/search/view_doc.asp?symbol=A/66/L.1.

24. De Maeseneer J, Roberts RG, et al. Tackling the NCDs: a different approach is needed. *Lancet* 378, no. 9791 (August 13, 2011).

25. Comment: Mobilising the world for chronic NCDs. *Lancet*, published online at www.thelancet.com, November 11, 2010, DOI:10.1016/S0140-6736(10)61891-0; Beaglehole R, Bonita R, et al. Priority actions for the non-communicable disease crisis. *Lancet* 377 (April 23, 2011): 1438–1447.

26. Lincoln P, Rundall P, et al. Conflicts of interest and the UN high-level meeting on non-communicable diseases. *Lancet* 378, no. 9804, (November 12, 2011): e6; Gale J and Stanford D. Nestle, Glaxo lobby UN over biggest "epidemic" battle since

AIDS. bloomberg.com, September 16, 2011; Deborah C. Will industry influence derail UN summit?, *BMJ* 343 (August 23, 2011):d5328.

27. This report was issued by the UN Secretary General in September 2012, based on an extensive WHO analysis of lessons learned from approaches to multisectoral partnerships that were relevant for strengthening the response to NCDs. The SG's report reviewed five models as options for global partnerships against NCDs: aligned independent efforts, social movements, a coordinated network, a loosely coordinated network around a social movement on NCDs, and a centralized formal partnership. See UN General Assembly. Note by the Secretary-General transmitting the report of the Director-General of the World Health Organization on options for strengthening and facilitating multisectoral action for the prevention and control of non-communicable diseases through effective partnership. 67th session, Item 114 of provisional agenda, document A/67/373, www.un.org/ga/search/view_doc.asp?symbol=A%2F67%2F373&Submit=Search&Lang=E. For private sector perspectives, see Hancock C, Kingo L, and Raynaud O. The private sector, international development and NCDs. *Globalization and Health* 7 (2011), 23; and Lohse N, Ersbøll C and Kingo L. Taking on the challenge of noncommunicable diseases: we all hold a piece of the puzzle. *International Journal of Gynecology and Obstetrics* 115, Suppl. 1 (2011): S52–S54.

28. Two Days in New York: Reflections on the UN NCD Summit. *Lancet Oncology* 12, no. 11 (October 2011): 981.

29. Collins PY, Insel TR, Chockalingam A, Daar A, and Maddox YT. Grand challenges in global mental health: integration in research, policy and practice. *PLoS Medicine.* 4 (April 10, 2013): e1001434; Becker AE and Kleinman A. Mental health and the global agenda. *New England Journal of Medicine* 369 (July 4, 2013): 66–73.

30. Bukhman G and Kidder A, eds. *The PIH Guide to Chronic Care Integration for Endemic Non-Communicable Diseases*, Rwanda Edition, Cardiac, Renal, Diabetes, Pulmonary and Palliative Care. Boston: Partners in Health, Harvard Medical School, Brigham and Women's Hospital, 2011; www.pih.org/library/the-pih-guide-to-chronic-care-integration-for-endemic-non-communicable-dise.

31. Anne G. World leaders agree to cut deaths from non-communicable diseases by a quarter by 2025. *BMJ* 344 (May 28, 2012): e3768; Beaglehole R, Bonita R, Horton R, et al. Measuring progress on NCDs: one goal and five targets. *Lancet* 380 (October 13, 2012): 1283–1285. See also Alleyne G, Binagwaho A, Haines A, Jahan S, Nugent R, Rojhani A, and Stuckler D. Embedding non-communicable diseases in the post-2015 development agenda. *Lancet* 381 (February 16, 2013): 566–574; and Horton R. Non-communicable diseases: 2015 to 2025. *Lancet* 381 (February 16, 2013): 509–510.

32. World Health Organization. Report of the Formal Meeting of Member States to conclude the work on the comprehensive global monitoring framework, including indicators, and a set of voluntary global targets for the prevention and

control of noncommunicable diseases. Document A/NCD/2, November 21, 2012, http://apps.who.int/gb/ncds/pdf/A_NCD_2-en.pdf; WHO. Revised (third) WHO Discussion Paper on the development of a comprehensive global monitoring framework, including indicators, and a set of voluntary global targets for the prevention and control of NCDs. 2013, www.who.int/nmh/events/2012/discussion _paper3.pdf.

33. World Health Organization. Draft action plan for the prevention and control of noncommunicable diseases, 2013–2020. Report by the Secretariat, 66th World Health Assembly, provisional agenda item 13.2, document A66/9, May 6, 2013, http://apps.who.int/gb/ebwha/pdf_files/WHA66/A66_9-en.pdf.

34. Ibid.; WHO. Draft comprehensive global monitoring framework and targets for the prevention and control of noncommunicable diseases. Report by the Director-General, 66th World Health Assembly, Provisional agenda item 13.1, document A66/8, March 15, 2013, http://apps.who.int/gb/ebwha/pdf_files/WHA66/A66_8-en .pdf.

35. Bollyky TJ, Noncommunicable diseases and the new global health, in Cahill KJ, ed., More with less: disasters in an era of diminishing resources. New York: Fordham University Press and the Center for International Humanitarian Cooperation, 2012, 95–109, esp. 109–109; Clark H. NCDs: a challenge to sustainable human development. *Lancet* 381 (February 16, 2013): 510–511; Alleyne G, Binagwaho A, Haines A, et al. Embedding non-communicable diseases in the post-2015 development agenda. *Lancet* 381 (February 16, 2013): 566–574; Frenk J and Moon S. Governance challenges in global health. *New England Journal of Medicine* 368 (March 7, 2013): 936–942; Berkley S, Chan M, Dybul M, et al. A healthy perspective: the post-2015 development agenda. *Lancet* 381 (March 30, 2013): 1076–1077; Thomas BP, Gostin LO. Tackling the global NCD crisis: innovations in law and governance. *Journal of Law, Medicine & Ethics* 41 (Spring 2013): 16–27; Task Team for the Global Thematic Consultation on Health in the Post-2015 Development Agenda. Health in the Post-2015 Agenda: Report of the Global Thematic Consultation on Health. New York: United Nations, April 2013.

36. Beaglehole R, Bonita R, Horton R. Independent global accountability for NCDs. *Lancet* 381 (February 23, 2013): 602–605; Bonita R, Magnusson R, Bovet P, et al. Country actions to meet UN commitments on non-communicable diseases: a stepwise approach. *Lancet* 381 (February 16, 2013): 575–584.

37. This regulation was struck down by the courts in March 2013; Grynbaum MM. Judge blocks New York City's limits on big sugary drinks. *New York Times*, March 11, 2013, www.nytimes.com/2013/03/12/nyregion/judge-invalidates-bloombergs-soda-ban.html?pagewanted=all&_r=0. See also Mariner WK and Annas GJ. Limiting "sugary drinks" to reduce obesity—who decides? *New England Journal of Medicine* 368 (May 9, 2013): 1763–1765;Fairchild A. Half empty or half full? New York's soda rule in historical perspective. *New England Journal of Medicine* 368 (May 9, 2013): 1765–1767.

38. Dowell D and Farley TA. Prevention of non-communicable diseases in New York City. *Lancet* 380 (November 17, 2012): 1787–1789.

39. Ibid.

40. Bloomberg Speaks on Non-Communicable Diseases at UN General Assembly. September 20, 2011, www.mikebloomberg.com/index.cfm?objectid=88C81DF6 -C29C-7CA2-FCBB0555D5B99541.

CHAPTER 1

Regulation of NCD Medicines in Low- and Middle-Income Countries

Current Challenges and Future Prospects

Brian White-Guay

The growing burden of noncommunicable diseases in low- and middle-income countries has highlighted the urgent need to improve access to essential drugs and technologies.[1] Considerable gaps remain, however, in the availability of essential medicines for acute and chronic conditions in LMICs, especially in Africa.

While the majority of countries have established national medicines regulatory authorities (NMRAs) responsible for reviewing and approving medicines, the level of available expertise and capability to fulfill all the essential functions of a regulatory authority often remain very limited.[2] This has led to delayed initiation of clinical trials and approval of medicines as well as increased circulation of substandard products. Many NMRAs have limited or no capabilities to enable effective measures of surveillance, to control NCD drugs' post-marketing experience, or to use promotional information. These problems are threatening to become even more troublesome as new efforts are mounted to deal with NCDs.

The recent initiatives aiming at promoting regional cooperation among NMRAs have thus become more important and will become even more significant as the NCD campaign gathers momentum. These initiatives include efforts to increase sharing of assessment expertise, to promote adoption of common technical standards, and to upgrade inspection activities. Improving access to medicines aimed at reducing the burden of NCDs will require greater support of regional cooperation schemes but also of appropriate convergence of structure and capacity building in NMRAs and the adoption of harmonized technical standards for registration across regions. This chapter reviews some of the current challenges and future prospects.

Regulatory Framework and Functions

Drug regulatory agencies worldwide share a common overall objective of protecting the public health by ensuring the efficacy, safety, manufacturing quality, and security of human medicinal products placed on their respective markets. The core elements of drug regulatory systems are closely related around the world, and the key attributes of effective regulatory programs have recently been reviewed.[3]

These core functions include licensing and inspection of manufacturing facilities and distribution channels, inspection of clinical trial sites and laboratories involved in the development of medicinal products, review and assessment of medicinal product marketing applications, control of drug promotion and advertising, review and oversight of clinical trials applications, and post-authorization pharmacovigilance and other risk-assessment, management, and communication activities.

The workload associated with these core activities is influenced by several factors, but it can be quite large and expensive, and costs will grow substantially as NCD treatment increases. Using the U.S. system as an example, the resources required to manage the human drugs and biologicals programs at the U.S. FDA was approximately US$ 1.2 billion, with close to 4,000 FTEs (full-time equivalents) in 2010.[4]

Such a level of support, which saw further significant increases in fiscal year 2012, is well beyond the reach of most NMRAs in the world. Thus, enabling core regulatory functions in most LMICs will need to be achieved in a gradual manner through certification of competency and the effective use of regional collaborations to leverage capabilities, resources, and expertise to meet public health needs associated with NCDs.

Several measures of performance can be used to assess process aspects of drug regulatory systems; these should include, at a minimum, efficiency, accountability,

---

Box 1.1 Certification Levels for National Medicines Regulatory Authorities

Level IV: An NRA competent and efficient in performing the regulatory functions as recommended by PAHO/WHO to assure efficacy, safety, and quality of medicines. Regulatory Authority of Reference for the Region.

Level III: An NRA competent and efficient that still needs to improve in the performance of certain regulatory functions as recommended by WHO/PAHO to assure efficacy, safety and quality of medicines.

Level II: Structures and/or organizations with the mandate of an NRA that comply with certain regulatory functions as recommended by WHO/PAHO to assure efficacy, safety and quality of medicines.

Level I: Health institutions that perform certain regulatory functions for medicines.

Sources: PAHO Resolution CD50R9. Di Fabio, JL. Drug and biologics regulatory systems in developing countries: core elements. Health systems based on primary health care. PAHO 2011, slide 13. www.iom.edu /~/media/Files/Activity%20Files/Global/RegulatoryCoreElements/Speaker%20Presentations/March%202 /DiFabo.pdf.

---

and transparency.[5] Fortunately, progress has been made by NMRAs in LMICs toward the establishment of a voluntary certification process that helps to identify the level of proficiency achieved in performance of core regulatory functions (box 1.1). Perhaps one of the most noteworthy examples comes from Latin America, following the adoption of a resolution to strengthen national regulatory authorities in the region.[6]

Nevertheless, abundant challenges remain. These will increase as already-overburdened NMRAs deal with the growing demands of organizing their NCD programs. Below, I review some of the current challenges faced by NMRAs in LMICs.

Licensing of Medicines

The complexity of activities required by drug regulatory agencies for the licensing of medicinal products is not well known by the public and often underappreciated by health professionals. Key attributes of robust regulatory systems that are universally recognized include: responsiveness, or the ability of an agency to maintain and expand its scientific knowledge base; an outcome-focused orientation, to ensure continuous monitoring of safety issues that can arise with both new and well-established products; rule-making that is clear and balanced for the particular regulated industry; proportional risk assessment, ensuring that any special requirements or limitations on use arising from a licensing decision are justified; and finally, independence and transparency.

Limited data are available on the total number of professional staff in NMRAs from LMICs, but both the number and the range of skills possessed by staff in these countries and needed to accomplish all regulatory functions are low. This has led to heavy workloads for individual staff members and long delays in reviewing marketing applications; as a result, a perception exists within the pharmaceutical industry of a significant burden of administrative requirements that are often duplicative among regulators within the same region. Of more concern is the fact that a recent study conducted in the sub-Saharan region concluded that the existing regulatory resources did not form a coherent regulatory system and that, on the whole, countries did not have the capacity to control the quality, safety, and efficacy of the medicines circulating on their markets.[7] Specific efforts have been made in recent years to improve access to treatments for neglected diseases, including some NCDs, and specific recommendations have been made in support of regulatory expertise and capacity building in particular to close these gaps, especially in the African region.[8]

Essential Medicines

Efforts to establish an essential medicines list (EML) to meet priority healthcare needs have been in place for over 30 years. Despite significant progress, the challenges to realizing the full promise of the EML have yet to be overcome.[9] In 2007, improved access to essential medicines for children was recognized as an important goal, and this has led to the creation of the first model EML for children.[10]

Whereas the first World Health Organization EML contained 216 molecules that included duplicates as well as 204 molecules that excluded duplicate listings, the most recent 2011 version of the WHO EML contains 445 medicines and 358 molecules, excluding duplicates.[11] If combined with the EML for children (EMLc), the total number is approximately 800 medicines for both adults and children. In contrast, the number of molecules, excluding duplicates, approved for human use by the U.S. FDA is estimated at 2,356, with an overall number of 10,000 products, including duplicates.[12] The total number of "drug products" (all dosages, forms, combinations and packs) registered by the FDA reaches a staggering figure of 100,000. The results of a 2007 WHO fact survey of 156 countries showed that 86% of responding countries had a national EML, including all low-income countries and most middle-income countries, and that the number of medicines included in the national EML varied, with a global median of 397.[13]

The third WHO Medicines Strategy has identified the need for both continuity and change in increasing global access to essential medicines.[14] Despite the progress made through collaboration with various stakeholders—including UN agencies involved in pharmaceutical program support, public-interest NGOs, research-based and generic pharmaceutical industries, and interested governmental and private donor organizations—there is an urgent need to close the availability gap identified in many countries.[15]

The WHO Prequalification of Medicines Program has been coordinating a novel quality risk assessment mechanism on behalf of the Global Fund to Fight AIDS, Tuberculosis and Malaria with the establishment of an Expert Review Panel (ERP). A recent review has shown that this process was well accepted by manufacturers and procurement agencies and that out of 115 eligible products assessed by the ERP in 2009 and 2010, 44 became prequalified or approved by a stringent authority thereafter.[16]

Procurement of quality medicines for evidence-based decision making based on stringent quality criteria for the provision of needed treatment options has proven effective for a number of essential medicines. The ERP advice, however, is not designed to ensure the continued compliance of manufacturers with stringent quality criteria standards on an ongoing basis, and as NCDs move to the forefront, there is an even greater need to link these efforts with the WHO prequalification program or other mechanisms to ensure periodic follow-up and requalification in the destination countries.

Improving access to essential medicines for the treatment of NCDs for a broader number of vulnerable patients thus continues to present a significant challenge. The availability of medicines for both acute and chronic conditions was found to be suboptimal across a recent survey in 40 developing countries, particularly in the public sector.[17] Availability of medicines for chronic conditions was lower than for acute conditions, suggesting that in efforts to improve management of NCDs, specific measures should be prioritized to improve access through concerned NMRAs from LMICs with the support of the WHO and international regulatory agencies.

Multisource Products

Increased access to quality generic products is an essential component of an overall strategy to improve the management of NCDs throughout the world. Generic pharmaceuticals represent almost two-thirds of total sales in low-income countries and about 60% of sales in middle-income countries. Branded generics are much more important than unbranded generics in terms of sales, but their higher cost can reduce their accessibility.

Some of the regulatory problems with NCD medicines might be eased by using the new FDA electronic drug listing system, which facilitates access to information regarding drug products, ingredients, firms, and facilities around the world, with the goal of improving the FDA's ability to screen imports of drugs at its borders efficiently and effectively. Clearly, the possibility of adapting such a system for other regions of the world would be invaluable to NMRAs in LMICs, but the funding and management of such a transnational system would have to be determined. Furthermore, current regulatory legislation, institutional frameworks, and capacities to regulate the movement of quality-assured medicines between countries remain quite disparate and an important obstacle to be addressed by the NCD campaign.[18] The recently updated second edition of the WHO's *Blue Book*, a manual for NMRAs on marketing authorization of multisource generic pharmaceutical products, provides practical guidance on regulatory requirements and procedures for handling NCD treatments, but its implementation will also require additional resources.[19]

NCD-focused regulatory tasks in LMICs will be lightened by the WHO certification scheme, another administrative tool developed in response to requests from WHO member states. This program was adopted in 1963 and has been updated continuously.[20] It is designed to help provide assurance of the quality, safety, and efficacy of pharmaceutical products imported by countries with limited regulatory capacity. Three types of certificates are issued under the scheme, namely a certificate of pharmaceutical product (CPP), a model batch certificate, and a model statement of the licensing status of a pharmaceutical product. The CPP provides information on the product to be registered in the importing country and the good manufacturing practice (GMP) status of the manufacturing plant—offering confirmation that it is the same as the one approved by the certifying country drug regulatory authority (DRA)—along with information about the reference DRA.

The goal is to provide a standard format for exchange of information between NMRAs through a harmonized procedure, which will facilitate timely access to medicines by making greater use of data generated by other qualified reference NMRAs. While problems remain in the implementation of the scheme,[21] the regulatory resource constraints in LMICs and the need to expand treatment options for NCDs should encourage expanded regional efforts toward adoption of harmonized registration requirements regarding CPPs. Significant progress toward this goal has been made in several regions in Africa, Asia, and especially Latin America, where advances have been spearheaded by the leadership of the Pan American Network for Drug Regulatory Harmonization.

Inspections and Quality Control

The increasing complexity that the NCD campaign will create for global supply chains (for both active pharmaceutical ingredients and finished products) will be a significant challenge for worldwide regulatory authorities. LMICs are already affected disproportionately by the problem of substandard and falsified medicines.[22] This concern has created an important global policy objective: to ensure consistency of approved product quality production standards and avoid fraud and other intentional adulteration of medicinal products entering international commerce.[23] A public health–oriented definition of poor-quality medicines has been proposed, which would include substandard, counterfeit, and degraded products together with a call for an international treaty on medicine quality.[24]

The Pharmaceutical Inspection Co-operation Scheme (PIC/S) is an international cooperation mechanism already firmly in place that should help to meet the NCD challenge. The pharmaceutical inspection authorities of 41 participating authorities from all regions are current members of this program. Its primary mission is to lead the international development, implementation, and maintenance of harmonized GMP standards and quality systems of inspectorates in the field of medicinal products. Industry representatives have called for greater use of mutual recognition agreements and/or Memoranda of Understanding to reduce the number of duplicative inspections by regulatory authorities around the world as well as greater focus on a risk-based approach to inspection and related processes. Industry has also called for increased acceptance of GMP certificates and CPPs prepared according to WHO recommendations and issued by competent regulatory authorities.

Few LMICs currently participate in the PIC/S because of membership accession requirements. The presence of the WHO as a partner organization to PIC/S does serve to ensure representation of their concerns and should be a basis for expanding and facilitating inspection capacity building and harmonization efforts with LMICs. Bringing more LMICs into the PIC/S should become a policy goal for the NCD movement.

Clinical Trials

Several problems with the conduct of clinical trials have been identified in LMICs, especially with respect to ethical considerations.[25] Significant barriers for NCD medicines include lack of the following: regulatory expertise and capacity in the review of clinical trials applications, authorization of importation of clinical batches, infrastructure for the conduct of studies, certification of researchers and research centers, training in the monitoring of good clinical practice (GCP), and funding mechanisms. The need to conduct multi-country studies further compounds these challenges. Regulatory pathways and procedures for clinical trials approval are often unclear and unpredictable, and sponsors may face substantial delays in trial initiation.

Three recent innovations provide encouragement to those working to improve NCD research, prevention, and treatment in LMICs. The creation of the African Vaccine Regulatory Forum in 2005 offers a model of an efficient, informal network for the regulation of vaccine clinical trials in Africa.[26] More recently, in 2009, the first Pan African Clinical Trials Registry[27] was established according to the criteria set up under the WHO for the International Clinical Trial Registry Platform. Finally, the recent creation of the Pan African Clinical Trial Alliance offers a new opportunity toward building harmonized procedures for GCP training, support for joint inspections, and review and ethical assessment of clinical trials.

Other, similar efforts are under way. In the Americas, the Pan American Health Organization (PAHO) established a working group of representatives from NMRAs in 1999 to implement harmonized GCP requirements in the region. The Asia-Pacific Economic Cooperation (APEC) Harmonization Center (AHC) has held three training workshops on multiregional clinical trials since 2009, with the aim of increasing convergence toward common procedures and practices in the Asia-Pacific region.[28] Strengthening of regulatory capacity in the area of clinical trials review and oversight through international and regional cooperation should be a core objective to improve access to, and treatment with, all medical products for NCDs.

Pharmacovigilance and Risk Management

The increased attention to drug safety concerns in industrialized countries has led to several recommendations aimed at reinforcing the structure of pharmacovigilance activities for both clinical trials and post-marketing follow-up for both new and well-established products.[29] Regulatory systems in LMICs have recognized the importance of building capacity in this area, and there is growing support through the WHO's International Conference of Drug Regulatory Authorities (ICDRA).

However, the number of LMICs with national pharmacovigilance systems registered with the WHO program for international drug monitoring remains quite limited, and increased access to medicines will not allow continuous monitoring of the risk-benefit profile in populations in these LMICs.[30] A high-priority area of concern for national pharmacovigilance systems in LMICs is to implement the capabilities programs to link falsified and substandard product reports to information on lack of efficacy to take corrective action. The new efforts to cope with NCDs should accelerate institutional change in pharmacovigilance.

The desirable goal of improving access through more efficient licensing procedures must be balanced with concerns about how these products will be used following their introduction to the market. This is a particular concern with NCD treatments, as it has been with the treatment of HIV infections.

Some of the considerations that point to the need for increased safety with use of well-established products that will be the primary treatments for NCDs include: unreliable supply chain systems for distribution, affecting quality and product performance; lack of trained healthcare workers who can advise on proper approved use and dosing information for patients; limited availability of treatment guidelines and information on risks for drug interactions; and a disproportionate representation of patients with low literacy levels and thus reduced ability to follow safety warnings for their medicines. Finally, concerns over long-term adherence to chronic therapy—which has been identified as a global issue, with LMIC rates even lower than the averages of 50% reported for developed countries—can be a problem, especially for patients on polypharmacy.[31] It is, of course, common for individual patients to require treatment for more than one NCD at a time, as these diseases are so often interrelated that contracting one type of NCD can increase the risk factors for others. Improving patient adherence is therefore a major NCD challenge.

As the NCD campaign gets under way, it is significant that several of the barriers to the promotion of pharmacovigilance in low- and middle-income NMRAs have already been identified, including the lack of adequate funding.[32] The importance of international collaboration in building capacity and training support in this field has been recognized and should benefit from the growing voluntary exchange agreements established between worldwide NMRAs, the WHO, and academic research centers. PAHO has sponsored the creation of specific regional guidance in this area, which represents a potential model for other regions.[33]

Good Governance of Medicines

The pharmaceutical sector has been recognized as highly vulnerable to corruption and unethical practices, thereby potentially further limiting the allocation of scarce health resources to increase access to good-quality essential medicines.[34] Furthermore, the integrity of administrative procedures in drug registration in developing countries has often been perceived negatively and as a business risk for pharmaceutical companies subject to global compliance requirements in their home jurisdictions. In 2009, the WHO established the Good Governance for Medicines (GGM) program, with the primary goal of reducing corruption in pharmaceutical systems through the application of transparency and accountability in all administrative procedures and the promotion of ethical practices.[35]

The NCD campaigns will require improved access to essential medicines—an integral part of a Global Health System (GHS) strategy. Four essential functions of governance for a GHS have been recently proposed: production of global public goods, management of externalities across countries, mobilization of global solidarity, and stewardship.[36] Efforts in support of regulatory systems convergence or harmonization and capacity-expertise building in LMICs that embody the GGM objectives *as well as* effectively support the broader framework of the GHS will ease the way toward expanded treatment for NCDs.

Regional Cooperation of NMRAs

New NCD campaigns will be able to build on the considerable efforts that have been made in the last decade in LMICs to foster greater cooperation between NMRAs from member states from different regional economic areas on all continents. With the support of the WHO, members of the ICH (International Conference on Harmonization of Technical Requirements for Registration of Pharmaceuticals for Human Use), other partner organizations, and some NGOs, foundations to further these efforts have been solidly established. Nevertheless, the gap between LMICs and high- and upper-income countries in terms of NMRA resources and capabilities remains large, and making investments to narrow it along a well-defined set of agreed priorities remains an important policy objective deserving of the attention and commitment of all concerned stakeholders.

Africa

The anticipated need for upgrading regulatory systems to prepare for more aggressive responses to NCDs is particularly acute in Africa. There are close to 50 NMRAs in Africa with substantial differences in registration, technical requirements, and administrative processes. As a result, manufacturers often target a limited set of countries for registration because of market size and entry barriers. A survey conducted by the Pharmaceutical Industry Association of South Africa (PIASA) identified several problems that contribute to limiting access.[37] Most notable are the inconsistent application of ICH guidelines, the lack of a common marketing application format, delayed registration timelines, country-specific packaging and labeling requirements, lack of mutual recognition of GMP inspections, elevated fees often seen as a revenue source, and, lastly, unpredictable post-registration requirements related to technical and safety variations.

Since 2009, the African Medicines Regulatory Harmonization (AMRH) initiative has worked toward building African capacity in all regulatory functions.[38] The model of support is widely based and includes both monetary and in-kind contributions, primarily in technical assistance from regulators and manufacturer organizations.

If convergence takes place as anticipated, approximately 5 to 10 Regional Economic Communities (RECs) will cooperate closely to manage NMRAs' support and development with common technical documentation, procedures, and decision-making frameworks. Meanwhile, efforts toward harmonization in the Southern African Development Community (SADC) have been continuing for several years, and recently the East Africa Community launched a similar program. The Economic Community of West African States has also been very active, adopting (in 2010) a common policy for human medicines regulation and establishing several working groups.[39] In light of the resolution adopted in 2011 by the Pan-African Parliament, other regions in Africa will likely follow suit in the near future.[40]

Additional international support has come from the World Bank (WB), which has developed an innovative arrangement wherein the Bank acts as the fund holder for pooled monies going into AMRH and other specific projects. The WB is cooperating with the New Partnership for Africa's Development, the WHO, the pharmaceutical industry, donors such as the Bill & Melinda Gates Foundation, other stakeholders, and RECs to ensure successful implementation and engagement across the continent.[41] Success with new coalitions of this sort will help establish the regulatory resources necessary for Africa's NCD campaign.

Asia-Pacific

Similar regulatory harmonization efforts are underway in the Asia-Pacific region. One, under the sponsorship of APEC, covers 21 countries, and the other, promoted by the Association of Southeast Asian Nations (ASEAN), includes 10 countries. APEC leaders established the life sciences innovation forum in 2002 and the regulatory harmonization initiative in 2008. In 2009, APEC followed with its Harmonization Center , utilized for standardizing regulatory processes for drugs and medical devices and as a coordinating center for training in these procedures and guidelines. To date, an overall strategic action plan has been developed and a multi-year planning cycle has been adopted. Progress toward convergence has been made in several areas, including multi-region clinical trials, good review practices, pharmaceutical quality standards, and pharmacovigilance.

Innovations in the ASEAN region will provide an improved institutional base for expansion in NCD treatment. The ASEAN region, established in 1967, has set a goal of putting in place an Asian Economic Community (AEC) by 2015, with a single market for goods, services, capital, and skilled labor. Following a policy decision on standards and conformance made in 2005, the organization issued, in 2009, guidance for the adoption of good regulatory practices aimed at achieving harmonization of technical standards and regulatory requirements under the pharmaceutical product working group. The initiative is well on the way to achieving its goals for regulatory harmonization in close cooperation with the WHO, ICH, APEC, and other partner organizations.

Latin America

Even more promising progress has been made in Latin America. The Pan American Network for Drug Regulatory Harmonization (PANDRH), which was established in 1999, covers 35 countries and 7 RECs in the Americas.[42] The member states have given full support to strengthening national regulatory authorities for medicines and biologicals and designating regulatory authorities of regional reference to participate in evaluation processes as part of PAHO's procurement mechanisms.[43] An assessment tool based on prior work done by the WHO has been developed to help regulatory authorities identify gaps in core functions and develop an appropriate institutional plan of action to achieve certification as a

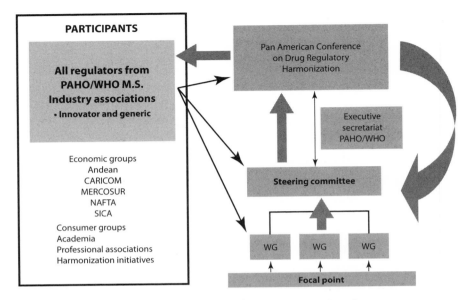

Fig. 1.1. Structure of the Pan American Conference on Drug Regulatory Harmonization. WG = (Technical) Working Group. Source: Pan American Network for Drug Regulatory Harmonization Statutes, Pan American Health Organization, www.paho.org.

reference NMRA with support for expertise development and capacity-building activities through PANDRH and PAHO partners. Currently, the overall structure of PANDRH provides for an integrated approach to regulatory harmonization and capacity building in the region, together with support for knowledge and experience transfer from the more-developed NMRAs to the less advanced. (See fig. 1.1.)

Accomplishments by working groups to date cover a very broad range of regulatory harmonization efforts in technical standards and requirements that cover most core regulatory functions:

- Good manufacturing practices
- Bioequivalence and bioavailability
- Good clinical practices
- Drug classification
- Counterfeit drugs
- Good laboratory practices
- Pharmacopeia

- Medicinal plants
- Drug registration
- Pharmacovigilance
- Vaccines and biotechnologicals
- Drug promotion

The progress in regulation in Latin America bodes well for NCD efforts and offers a good example of the benefits of cooperation between more developed and less developed agencies for complex product applications.[44] Global as well as regional harmonization efforts are promising even though the added burden of NCD medicines is anticipated. Greater support for interregional cooperation will truly help to fulfill the vision of an integrated global regulatory network.

ICH

Almost a decade after its successful launch in the member regions, in 1999 the International Conference on Harmonization of Technical Requirements for Registration of Pharmaceuticals for Human Use (ICH) created the Global Cooperation Group (GCG); this group's purpose is to establish more global links with countries outside the three ICH founding regions that were interested in learning more about the guidelines and the ICH process. Subsequently, in 2003, in recognition of the increased interest of regions with Regional Harmonization Initiatives (RHIs) that were determined to better understand and apply the guidance, a new partnership was established, with RHI representatives invited to participate in ICH technical discussions.

The GCG meetings offer an opportunity for RHI representatives to communicate requests for training and support for the dissemination of information on ICH guidelines in their region. Currently, the RHIs represented include APEC, ASEAN, the Gulf Cooperation Council (GCC), PANDRH, and SADC as well as NMRAs from the following countries: Australia, Brazil, China, Taipei, India, South Korea, Russia, and Singapore. Meetings of the ICH Global Cooperation Group take place during regular biannual ICH gatherings. These meetings enable RHIs and NMRAs to discuss specific ICH topics with technical experts present for the regular ICH conference.

In 2007 ICH created a Regulators Forum to increase the participation of individual NMRAs that were a major source of active pharmaceutical ingredients (API) or clinical trial data and those that had adopted ICH guidelines. The ICH operating principles state that it does not impose its views on any NMRA and that the GCG should work in close cooperation with the WHO and other international organizations involved in drug registration activities.

The benefits of advancing regulatory harmonization in support of public health in the ICH founding regions have been well recognized,[45] and the NCD campaign will make those benefits even more important. But to date, ICH has focused primarily on new chemical and biological substances and new dosage forms that contain new substances rather than on the well-established generics that form the backbone of much NCD treatment. The challenge of pursuing harmonization in areas that are more relevant to the NCD needs of less-developed regions has not yet been fully met.

The World Health Organization

From its inception in 1946, the WHO charter specifically recognized its role of developing, establishing, and promoting international standards with respect to food, biologics, and pharmaceutical products. A complete description of the contributions of the WHO in support of regulatory training and capacity building in LMICs and global harmonization efforts in the pharmaceutical sector is beyond the scope of this chapter, but several important accomplishments include the Essential Medicines List (EML), the International Nonproprietary Names, the International Pharmacopeias, the International Drug Pharmacovigilance program, good manufacturing practices, (GMP) and good clinical practice (GCP) as well as technical standards and guidelines for the pharmaceutical development and approval of the multisource generic products that will play a central role in expanded NCD treatment.

In response to the need expressed by United Nations agencies (which were purchasing these products) to make quality priority medicines available for reproductive health and for diseases such as HIV, malaria, and tuberculosis, in 2001 the WHO established a prequalification program in collaboration with NMRAs and partner organizations. The primary objectives were to apply uniform standards; conduct a comprehensive assessment of quality, efficacy, and safety of medicinal products; and prequalify quality control laboratories so that UN agencies could make better-informed product purchasing decisions. The prequalification program has also served to launch a capacity-building effort to provide staff from NMRAs with specially designed training in quality assessment, inspection of manufacturing sites, and prequalification of quality control laboratories for pharmaceuticals. According to the most recent Level I WHO indicator survey,[46] 50% of middle-income and 70% of low-income countries report using the prequalification scheme.

In the area of regulatory systems, the WHO has sponsored a biennial International Conference of Drug Regulatory Authorities since 1980, with the goal of improving regulatory harmonization and promoting exchange of information between NMRAs facing similar issues arising from global trade, new technologies, and e-commerce. Finally, the WHO has also been involved in the development of tools to assess the regulatory capacity of NMRAs and to provide appropriate technical support and training to address the gaps identified.[47] In all these ways, the WHO has proved central to improving global, regional, and national regulatory capacities, and it will need to continue such leadership by serving as a central actor in the NCD campaign.

Discussion

A study of the volume of medicines used to treat chronic diseases in the nonhospital sector across different WHO country income categories between 1997 and 2008 shows an important gap between high- (80%) and low-middle income (60%) countries, with roughly 35% of these medicines being listed on the WHO essential medicines list of 2007, irrespective of income categories.[48] This study targets the gap the NCD initiative seeks to close. While progress has been made in improving regulatory policies, NCDs create new and difficult problems. With respect to the four main NCDs—cardiovascular diseases (CVDs), diabetes, cancer, and chronic respiratory diseases—efforts to improve prevention measures along with access to essential medicines will have to be prioritized to focus on high-risk individuals.[49]

Regulatory systems constraints in LMICs currently limit access to essential medicines, especially quality-assured versions of these medicines, for treatment of both communicable and noncommunicable diseases. Few NMRAs in LMICs can support and fully manage all core regulatory functions on their own; this further affects the timely review of new submissions for approval, clinical trials, and pharmacovigilance and inspection activities within their jurisdictions. The major regulatory barriers include lack of: overall capacity, available expertise, information systems support, and formal cooperation agreements within some regions and with stringent regulatory agencies (SRAs). Cooperation can facilitate reliance on information and work done by other NMRAs, cut back on duplicative or redundant administrative requirements, and deal with insufficient funding mechanisms and delayed implementation of good governance practices.

A shared end-stage vision of what regulatory convergence efforts should be aiming to create is needed. Although regulatory cooperation has progressed significantly over the last 10 to 15 years in non-ICH countries, there is a considerable range in the scope of declared regulatory goals and interests in RECs, ranging from voluntary cooperation to the establishment of a single market of sovereign member states within a region. In the latter case, full harmonization of regulatory systems, procedures, and technical requirements is a prerequisite and can take time to achieve. The WHO Package of Essential Noncommunicable Disease Interventions (PEN) published in 2010 offers a conceptual framework to integrate reforms and improve measures to lower the burden of NCDs in low-resource settings.[50] Regulatory convergence efforts should be aligned in support of these efforts.

The key question is: what are the priority areas of regulatory convergence required to improve access to essential medicines for NCDs? The NCD campaign must address four main areas.

First is an effort to ensure that the approved medicines meet GMP specifications for high quality. This needs to be determined by a thorough review of submitted applications for multisource products, by inspections of manufacturing facilities by competent authorities, and by appropriate quality control measures of wholesalers / distribution networks and retail distributors. In light of its primary duties as a standard-setting organization and provider of scientific expertise and consensus, the WHO recently proposed the establishment of a global network of NMRAs in LMICs,[51] with a goal of gradually transferring the responsibility for prequalification of medicines from the WHO to this network (with an initial focus on prequalifying essential generic medicines for both adults and children based on uniform quality standards). This represents a welcome opportunity to devolve prequalification responsibilities at the appropriate national responsibility level through a cooperative effort to mobilize expertise and resources.

Second is the effort to ensure that access to EMLs is facilitated by supporting NMRAs, especially in low-income countries that fall short of this goal because of insufficient capacity, expertise, or funding.

Third will be improving access to and use of EMLs for the management of NCDs. This will require several coordinated measures from the national health care systems, such as regularly updated standard treatment guidelines and education on rational use by health care professionals and health assistants as well as others who come under the core regulatory functions of NMRAs. These policies include but are not limited to releasing regularly updated information on safety and efficacy for registered products, exerting controls over inappropriate promotion practices, and establishing effective capabilities in pharmacovigilance and risk communication. Novel approaches will be required to ensure that over time, the purported benefit-risk profile of products initially assessed in other more-developed settings will be extended within the setting of intended uses in LMICs to help lower the burden of NCDs.

Fourth is the improvement of capabilities and expertise for the timely review and oversight of clinical trials conducted in LMICs. At a minimum, more explicit regulatory convergence objectives related to these four priorities are needed in LMICs, especially in response to the globalization of medicines development and supply chains and the need to ensure access to quality-controlled medicines in a timely manner. The current sources of public, private, and NGO support for building regulatory capacity and expertise in LMICs remain fragmented and limited by institutional mandates. The NCD initiative would clearly gain from a more coherent global framework of coordination and execution that could subsequently promote networks of collaboration for the adoption of harmonized technical norms and standards.

The path to greater regulatory convergence of NMRAs and to a Level III or IV certification of competence (PAHO/WHO) has been well marked out in Latin America and Asia, but the situation in Africa calls for a better coordinated approach to policies promoting harmonization. Full harmonization of regulatory systems may be a worthwhile goal for some regions, but it is not a prerequisite for progress against NCDs.

The recent global financial crisis has had a direct impact on the availability of funds for health interventions in developing countries,[52] and this has led in turn to an increased call for accessibility and transparency of development aid for health spending from both public and private channels.[53] There is currently limited transparency in financial aid efforts to build regulatory resources in each region. Recent discussions around the funding dialogue proposals for the WHO have highlighted the importance of priority setting and program coherence.[54]

Successful regulatory reform and capacity building with NCDs in mind will create new demands for priority setting by concerned member states, with the expert and technical support of the WHO, the World Bank (e.g., AMRH), and

SRAs. Monetary and nonmonetary sources of support for reform can come from governments, NGOs, and industry through an appropriately designed and managed collaborative funding effort for each region.

Conclusion

National systems for regulating medicines have benefited in recent years from the increased cooperation in different regions of the world and the convergence toward the development of common technical standards based on ICH. But more should be done to adapt these standards to the priority needs of LMICs. Multisectoral action will be needed to achieve key public health objectives and lower the growing burden of NCDs in LMICs. Improved national and regional regulatory systems for medicines can contribute to the achievement of these goals.

The recommendations for action in support of the NCD campaign are:

- Develop an end-stage vision for desired regulatory convergence efforts. Develop a common vision for the regulatory systems of NMRAs in each RHI based on the most urgent priorities to improve access to high-quality essential medicines. Identify intermediate results indicators for the achievement of desired objectives. Review regulatory systems development proposals within each REC to gain member states' full endorsement and support for their chosen proposal's execution over a defined time period.
- Identify national and stakeholder funding models to support realization. Expand innovative stakeholders' funding and execution support mechanisms, such as that established with the World Bank in support of the AMRH initiative. Improve coordination of industry support efforts, which are currently still too fragmented and focused on product acceptance or isolated disease franchise support.
- Improve coordination of training and capacity building efforts. Fund a research proposal under WHO sponsorship to obtain Level III indicators of regulatory systems and provide an updated comprehensive review and gap analysis of core regulatory functions capacity and systems in LMICs. Expand ICH/WHO support to facilitate the adoption of existing guidelines and the development of guidelines for technical harmonization priorities in LMICs. Expand clinical trials registration and scientific

assessment support efforts in LMICs for the assessment and monitoring of clinical trials through RHI-coordinated plans with SRA support, including access to a common searchable database for ongoing studies. Improve coordination of SRAs, academe, the pharmaceutical industry, and NGOs for training efforts aimed at strengthening regulatory capacity and good governance. Improve overall NMRA transparency by improving access to WHO public assessment reports, WHO public inspection reports, and other important alerts and communications concerning the safe use of approved medicines.

- Improve regional cooperation efforts and information exchange platforms. Identify current best practices for core regulatory functions across RHIs and facilitate their assessment and transfer through a process supported by the WHO or others. Identify management practices and efficient administrative procedures that can reduce inefficiency and the waste of limited resources in NMRAs. Support the establishment of a fully operational and funded network of quality control laboratories to limit circulation of substandard or counterfeit medicines. Establish a secure exchange e-platform to facilitate communications and knowledge transfer between NMRAs from LMICs and SRAs. Using models from the United States and the EU, develop access to database systems on manufacturing licenses, import authorizations, and GMP certificates adapted to product applications for NMRAs in LMICs.

As the NCD movement acts and advocates to establish these improved regulatory policies, it will help to ensure that NCD patients in LMICs gain better access to more reliable and higher-quality health products vital to their well-being. In this way, we can begin to turn the tide in the battle against the global NCD epidemic.

NOTES

I wish to thank the following people for their suggestions on the approach for this work and their useful advice: Vincent Ahonkhai, BMGF; Emer Cooke, EMA; Mike Ward, Health Canada; Elaine Whiting, AstraZeneca UK Ltd. This chapter has been reviewed in draft form by individuals with diverse perspectives and technical expertise. I thank the following colleagues for their candid and critical comments: James

Fitzgerald, Pan American Health Organization; Peter Honig, AstraZeneca Pharmaceuticals; Murray M. Lumpkin, U.S. Food and Drug Administration; Tonya L. Villafana, World Bank. Responsibility for the final content of this chapter rests entirely with the author.

1. Beaglehole R, Bonita R, Alleyne G, Horton R, Li L, Lincoln P, et al. UN High-level Meeting on Non-communicable Diseases: addressing four questions. *Lancet.* 2011 Jul 30;378(9789):449–55. PubMed PMID: 21665266. Epub 2011/06/15; WHO. Global Status Report on Noncommunicable Diseases. Geneva: WHO, 2011; Alwan A, Maclean DR, Riley LM, d'Espaignet ET, Mathers CD, Stevens GA, et al. Monitoring and surveillance of chronic non-communicable diseases: progress and capacity in high-burden countries. *Lancet.* 2010 Nov 27;376(9755):1861–8. PubMed PMID: 21074258.

2. Assessment of medicines regulatory systems in sub-Saharan African countries. Geneva: WHO, 2010.

3. Ensuring safe foods and medical products through stronger regulatory systems abroad. Washington, DC: Institute of Medicine, 2012.

4. U.S. Department of Health and Social Security. The Food and Drug Administration's congressional justification. 2012, p. 622.

5. Ratanawijitrasin S, Wondemagegnehu E. Effective drug regulation: a multi-country study. Geneva: WHO, 2002.

6. Pan American Health Organization. Strengthening national regulatory authorities for medicines and biologicals. CD50.R9. PAHO, 2010.

7. World Health Organization. Assessment of medicines regulatory systems in sub-Saharan African countries. Geneva: WHO, 2010.

8. Moran M, Strub-Wourgaft N, Guzman J, Boulet P, Wu L, Pecoul B. Registering new drugs for low-income countries: the African challenge. *PLoS medicine.* 2011 Feb;8(2):e1000411. PubMed PMID: 21408102. Pubmed Central PMCID: 3051317. Epub 2011/03/17.

9. Robertson J, Hill SR. The essential medicines list for a global patient population. *Clinical pharmacology and therapeutics.* 2007 Nov;82(5):498–500. PubMed PMID: 17952104.

10. Zucker H, Rago L. Access to essential medicines for children: the world health organization's global response. *Clinical pharmacology and therapeutics.* 2007 Nov;82(5):503–5. PubMed PMID: 17952106. Epub 2007/10/24.

11. World Health Organization. The world medicines situation 2011—selection of essential medicines. Geneva: WHO, 2011.

12. Huang R, Southall N, Wang Y, Yasgar A, Shinn P, Jadhav A, et al. The NCGC pharmaceutical collection: a comprehensive resource of clinically approved drugs enabling repurposing and chemical genomics. *Science translational medicine.* 2011 Apr 27;3(80):80ps16. PubMed PMID: 21525397. Pubmed Central PMCID: 3098042.

13. WHO. Country pharmaceutical situations. Fact book on WHO Level I indicators. Geneva: WHO, 2007.

14. WHO. Implementing the third WHO medicines strategy 2008–2013. WHO, 2009.

15. Mendis S, Fukino K, Cameron A, Laing R, Filipe A, Jr., Khatib O, et al. The availability and affordability of selected essential medicines for chronic diseases in six low- and middle-income countries. *Bull World Health Organ.* 2007 Apr;85(4):279–88. PubMed PMID: 17546309. Pubmed Central PMCID: 2636320. Epub 2007/06/05.

16. WHO Prequalification of Medicines Programme. *WHO Drug Information* 2012;26(2):99–108.

17. Cameron A, Roubos I, Ewen M, Mantel-Teeuwisse AK, Leufkens HG, Laing RO. Differences in the availability of medicines for chronic and acute conditions in the public and private sectors of developing countries. *Bull World Health Organ.* 2011 Jun 1;89(6):412–21. PubMed PMID: 21673857. Pubmed Central PMCID: 3099556. Epub 2011/06/16.

18. Chen ML, Shah VP, Crommelin DJ, Shargel L, Bashaw D, Bhatti M, et al. Harmonization of regulatory approaches for evaluating therapeutic equivalence and interchangeability of multisource drug products: workshop summary report. *Eur J Pharm Sci.* 2011 Nov 20;44(4):506–13. PubMed PMID: 21946259. Epub 2011/09/29.

19. WHO Division of Drug Management and Policies. Marketing authorization of pharmaceutical products with special reference to multisource (generic) products: a manual for National Medicines Regulatory Authorities (NMRAs). 2nd edition. Geneva: WHO, 2011.

20. WHO. Certification Scheme on the Quality of Pharmaceutical Products Moving in International Commerce. Accessed September 14, 2012. www.who.int/medicines/areas/quality_safety/regulation_legislation/certification/en/index.html.

21. Whitting E. How has the evolution of the global pharmaceutical market affected the use of Certificates of Pharmaceutical Product (CPP)? *Regulatory Rapporteur.* 2012;9(4):8–11.

22. Institute of Medicine. Countering the problem of falsified and substandard drugs. Washington, DC: IOM. National Academies Press, 2013.

23. U.S. Food and Drug Administration. Pathway to global product safety and quality. A special report. U.S. FDA, 2011.

24. Newton PN, Amin AA, Bird C, Passmore P, Dukes G, Tomson G, et al. The primacy of public health considerations in defining poor quality medicines. *PLoS medicine.* 2011 Dec;8(12):e1001139. PubMed PMID: 22162953. Pubmed Central PMCID: 3232210. Epub 2011/12/14; Attaran A, Barry D, Basheer S, Bate R, et al. How to achieve international action on falsified and substandard medicines. *BMJ* 2012 Nov;345:e7381.

25. Caplan AL. Clinical trials of drugs and vaccines among the desperately poor in poor nations: ethical challenges and ethical solutions. *Clinical pharmacology and therapeutics.* 2010 Nov;88(5):583–4. PubMed PMID: 20959841.

26. World Health Organization, ed. Fifth Meeting of the African Vaccine Regulatory Forum (AVAREF). Final Report. Nairobi, Kenya, 2010. www.who.int/immunization_standards/vaccine_regulation/avaref5_report_nairobi_2010.pdf.

27. Abrams AL. One of a kind—the Pan African Clinical Trials Registry, a regional registry for Africa. *Pan African Medical Journal*. 2011;9(42):195–200. www.panafrican-med-journal.com/content/article/9/42/full/.

28. Park KL, Kim TG, Seong SK, Lee SY, Kim SH. APEC Harmonization Center: challenges and issues relating to multiregional clinical trials in the APEC region. *Clinical pharmacology and therapeutics*. 2012 Apr;91(4):743–6. PubMed PMID: 22318621. Epub 2012/02/10.

29. Baciu A, Stratton, K, Burke SP. The future of drug safety: promoting and protecting the health of the public. Washington, DC: National Academies Press, 2007.

30. Pirmohamed M, Atuah KN, Dodoo AN, Winstanley P. Pharmacovigilance in developing countries. *BMJ*. 2007 Sep 8;335(7618):462. PubMed PMID: 17823149. Pubmed Central PMCID: 1971195. Epub 2007/09/08.

31. World Health Organization. Adherence to long-term therapy: evidence for action. Geneva: WHO, 2003. www.who.int/chp/knowledge/publications/adherence_full_report.pdf.

32. Olsson S, Pal SN, Stergachis A, Couper M. Pharmacovigilance activities in 55 low- and middle-income countries: a questionnaire-based analysis. *Drug Saf*. 2010 Aug 1;33(8):689–703. PubMed PMID: 20635827. Epub 2010/07/20; Stergachis A, Bartlein RJ, Dodoo A, Nwokike J, Kachur SP. A situational analysis of pharmacovigilance plans in the Global Fund Malaria and U.S. President's Malaria Initiative proposals. *Malaria journal*. 2010;9:148. PubMed PMID: 20509971. Pubmed Central PMCID: 2887883.

33. Pan American Health Organization. Good pharmacovigilance practices for the Americas. Working Group on Pharmacovigilance, PANDRH Technical Document No. 5. Washington, DC: PAHO, 2011. http://apps.who.int/medicinedocs/documents/s18625en/s18625en.pdf.

34. Cohen JC, Mrazek M, Hawkins L. Tackling corruption in the pharmaceutical systems worldwide with courage and conviction. *Clinical pharmacology and therapeutics*. 2007 Mar;81(3):445–9. PubMed PMID: 17251983.

35. World Health Organization. A framework for good governance in the pharmaceutical sector. Working draft for field testing and revision, October 2008. Geneva: WHO, 2009. www.who.int/medicines/areas/policy/goodgovernance/GGM-framework09.pdf.

36. Frenk J, Moon S. Governance challenges in global health. *N Engl J Med*. 2013 Mar 7;368(10):936–42. PubMed PMID: 23465103.

37. Narsai K. Impact of regulatory requirements on medicines access in African countries. Pharmaceutical Industry Association of South Africa, 2010. www.piasa.co.za.

38. Ndomondo-Sigonda M, Ambali A. The African medicines regulatory harmonization initiative: rationale and benefits. *Clinical pharmacology and therapeutics*. 2011 Feb;89(2):176–8. PubMed PMID: 21252936. Epub 2011/01/22.

39. UEMOA (West African Economic and Monetary Union). Règlement 06/2010 /CM/UEMOA Relatif aux procédures d'homologation des produits pharmaceutiques

à usage humain dans les etats membres de l'UEMOA. June 2010. www.uemoa.int /Documents/Actes/Reg_06_2010_CM_UEMOA.pdf.

40. Pan-African Parliament. Recommendations and resolutions of the committee on health, labour and social affairs on the African medicines registration harmonisation initiative. Midrand, South Africa: May 2011. www.pan-africanparliament .org/DocumentsResources_DisplayDocument.aspx?Type=Docs&ID=1230.

41. African Medicines Regulatory Harmonization. Proceedings of the African Medicines Regulatory Harmonization (AMRH) stakeholders' plenary consultation meeting, Arusha, Tanzania. March 29, 2012. www.amrh.org/sites/default/files/down loads/amrh_meeting_20120329_proceedings_final_draft.pdf.

42. Pan American Network for Drug Regulatory Harmonization webpage. PAHO. http://new.paho.org/hq/index.php?option=com_content&view=category&layout=blog &id=1156&Itemid=513&lang=en.

43. Pan American Health Organization. Strenghtening national regulatory authorities for medicines and biologicals. PAHO CD50.R9, 2010. http://iris.paho.org /xmlui/bitstream/handle/123456789/427/CD50.R9-e.pdf?sequence=1.

44. Pombo ML, Di Fabio JL, Cortes Mde L. Review of regulation of biological and biotechnological products in Latin American and Caribbean countries. *Biologicals*. 2009 Oct;37(5):271–6. PubMed PMID: 19664935. Epub 2009/08/12.

45. Molzon JA, Giaquinto A, Lindstrom L, Tominaga T, Ward M, Doerr P, et al. The value and benefits of the International Conference on Harmonisation to drug regulatory authorities: advancing harmonization for better public health. *Clinical pharmacology and therapeutics*. 2011 Apr;89(4):503–12. PubMed PMID: 21326288. Epub 2011/02/18.

46. World Health Organization. Country pharmaceutical situations. Fact book on Level I indicators 2007. Geneva: WHO, 2011.

47. WHO data collection tool for the review of drug regulatory systems. WHO /TCM/MRS/2007.1. Geneva: WHO, 2007. www.who.int/medicines/areas/quality _safety/regulation_legislation/ENdatacollectiontool.pdf.

48. World Health Organization. The world medicines situtation 2011: pharmaceutical consumption. Geneva: WHO, 2011.

49. Beaglehole R, Bonita R, Horton R, Ezzati M, Bhala N, Amuyunzu-Nyamongo M, et al. Measuring progress on NCDs: one goal and five targets. *Lancet*. 2012 Oct 13;380(9850):1283–5. PubMed PMID: 23063272.

50. World Health Organization. Package of essential noncommunicable (PEN) disease interventions for primary health care in low-resource settings. Geneva: WHO, 2010, p. 65.

51. World Health Organization. Regulator prequalification of medicines: a future concept for networking. *WHO Drug Information* 2012 2(3):239–246.

52. Leach-Kemon K, Chou DP, Schneider MT, Tardif A, Dieleman JL, Brooks BP, et al. The global financial crisis has led to a slowdown in growth of funding to improve health in many developing countries. *Health Aff (Millwood)*. 2012 Jan;31(1):228–35. PubMed PMID: 22174301.

53. Grepin KA, Leach-Kemon K, Schneider M, Sridhar D. How to do (or not to do) . . . tracking data on development assistance for health. *Health Policy Plan.* 2012 Sep;27(6):527–34. PubMed PMID: 22155590.

54. Legge D. Future of WHO hangs in the balance. *BMJ.* 2012;345:e6877. PubMed PMID: 23100330.

CHAPTER 2

Improving Access to Medicines for Noncommunicable Diseases through Better Supply Chains

Lisa Smith and Prashant Yadav

Priority noncommunicable diseases,[1] such as diabetes, cardiovascular diseases, chronic respiratory diseases, and cancers, represent a large portion of the total global morbidity and mortality. Noncommunicable diseases in low- and middle-income countries account for 80% of the total global burden of NCDs.[2] Current projections estimate that the total share of deaths attributable to NCDs will rise by 50% in low- and middle-income countries by 2030.[3] In addition to this increasing burden, many low- and middle-income countries face a dual burden of disease where communicable diseases (CDs), such as malaria and tuberculosis, remain prevalent while at the same time, individuals are increasingly impacted by NCDs. NCDs in low- and middle-income countries, as compared to high-income countries, affect local economies at earlier stages in development, with fewer available resources to address them as well as varying degrees of health system infrastructure to support appropriate care. Multisectoral policies aimed at decreasing risk factors and increasing effective and affordable delivery of health sector interventions are needed to achieve the global goals of 25% reduction in premature mortality due to NCDs by 2025.[4]

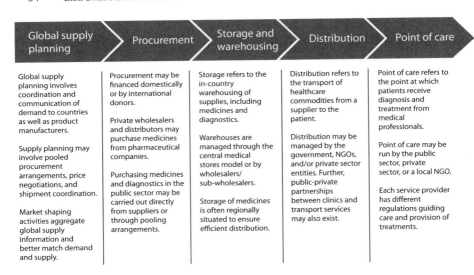

Fig. 2.1. Typical supply chain structure.

Delivery and provision of care for noncommunicable diseases requires ongoing access to a diverse set of medicines, consistent adherence to treatment regimes, and use of diagnostics, which vary in complexity, for management of each disease. Improved access to NCD medicines requires a well-functioning supply chain that delivers these medicines to the end population affordably and in an equitable manner. Well-functioning supply chains require global coordination and extensive planning of procurement, storage, distribution, and point-of-care dispensing. Currently, the functional and structural organization of the global supply chain for NCD medicines is far from optimal. (See fig. 2.1.)

In addition to complexities in the overall medicines supply chain, supply chains for NCD medicines have to cater to certain unique considerations such as a greater number of required treatments and diagnostics / management tools, ongoing treatment and disease management, and increased levels of training and involvement of medical professionals. Improving access to NCD medicines requires a thorough understanding of the structural obstacles in medicine supply chains as well as a holistic rethinking of access and integration of care from the top of the supply chain down to the patient / point of care. The process of rethinking access and service delivery for NCDs has already begun in several forums. The NCD Alliance and the World Health Organization have adopted access to NCD medicines as a central advocacy effort.[5] This chapter examines gaps in research on, and practice of, supply and distribution planning that limit access to NCD medicines as well as develops recommendations for improvement.

Role of Medicines and Technologies in Noncommunicable Diseases

Comprehensive solutions that involve strengthening health systems, increasing financing for noncommunicable diseases, better training of healthcare workers, and improved access to medicines are all needed to address NCDs in developing countries. In this section we highlight the role of improving access to medicines and specific preventive technologies for NCDs as well as factors that currently inhibit increased access to medicines.

Priority Medicines for Noncommunicable Diseases

The prevention and treatment of NCDs is directly dependent on access to preventive technologies and medicines. While access to preventive technologies is important, this paper focuses on improvements in access to medicines and specific medical devices for NCDs.

The spectrum of medicines used to treat noncommunicable diseases is wide, with multiple treatments for each disease area. Table 2.1 lists the medicines included on the essential medicines list as developed by the World Health Organization, but this list does not include all available medicines of quality or substandard quality that are available to individuals.

Factors that Inhibit Access to NCD Medicines

The global target for availability of essential medicines and technologies, including generics, used to treat major NCDs in both public and private facilities is set at 80%.[6] However, in many low- and middle-income countries access to NCD medicines remains severely limited due to a combination of factors.

Lack of Affordability

In most low-income countries and some lower-middle-income countries, affordability of NCD medicines remains a constraint for many individuals with noncommunicable diseases. The long-term management of NCDs requires long periods of purchasing treatments, which may mean a larger financial burden for

Table 2.1 Non-cancer WHO Essential Medicines List for noncommunicable diseases

	Drug category	Active ingredient	Available as generic
Asthma/COPD	Short-activating beta-agonists	Epinephrine	Yes
	Long-acting beta-agonists	Salbutamol	Yes
	Inhaled corticosteroids	Beclometasone	Yes[a]
		Budesonide	Yes[a]
	Vagolytics	Ipratropium	Yes
	Systemic corticosteroids	Prednisolone	Yes
		Dexamethasone	Yes
Coronary artery disease	Anti-platelet drugs	Acetylsalicylic acid	Yes
	Nitrates	Glyceryl trinitrate	Yes
		Isosorbide dinitrate	Yes
	Beta-blockers	Bisoprolol	Yes
	Lipid-lowering drugs	Simvastatin	Yes
	Calcium channel blockers	Verapamil	Yes
		Amlodipine	Yes
	Other antihypertensives	Methyldopa	Yes
Congestive heart failure	Diuretics	Hydrochlorothiazide	Yes
		Furosemide	Yes
		Amiloride	Yes
		Spironolactone	Yes
	ACE inhibitors	Enalapril	Yes
	Anticoagulants	Warfarin	Yes
	Inotropic agents	Digoxin	Yes
	Other vasodilators	Hydralazine	Yes
Diabetes	Oral hypoglycemic	Glibenclamide	Yes
		Metformin	Yes
	Short-acting insulin	Various	Yes[b]
	Depot insulin	Various	Yes[b]
	Insulin antagonists	Glucagon	Yes

Source: RAND review of WHO EML. Mattke S, Haims M, Ayivi-Guedehoussou N, Gillen E, Hunter L, Klautzer L, and Mengistu T. Improving access to medicines for non-communicable diseases in the developing world. RAND Health, 2011. www.rand.org/pubs/occasional_papers/OP349.html.

[a] While inhaled steroids as active ingredients are no longer protected by patent, some delivery technologies for the inhalers are still protected.

[b] Several insulin products have lost their patent protection, but others are still protected. The availability of biosimilar insulin products in a given jurisdiction depends on its regulatory framework for biosimilars.

individuals over prolonged periods of time. In addition, many individuals have to pay for the treatment of multiple chronic conditions at the same time, as NCDs are often caused by similar social determinants and exposure to related risk factors.[7] Further, the shared risk factors and increasing connection between NCDs and CDs means that management of comorbidities is increasingly common. As a result of these factors and the high percentage of out-of-pocket healthcare expenditures, nonfunctioning supply chains remain a key factor influencing affordability of medicines.

With varying availability and few public or private sector healthcare insurance options, an individual's ability and willingness to pay for products determines the overall demand. In many low- and middle-income countries, out-of-pocket expenditures account for up to 50% of total healthcare costs.[8] Often when medicines are out of stock in the public sector clinics, patients purchase medicines in the private sector, where prices are much higher. The financial burden of NCD treatments on patients may force individuals to purchase medicines in suboptimal ways. Examining 14 high-burden NCD medicines across 24 low- and middle-income countries, median days' wages for NCD medicines varied considerably by disease type and country.[9] For glibenclamide, a diabetes medicine, affordability ranged between 0.2 days' wages and 8.3 days' wages for a 30-day supply of 1 tablet taken twice daily. Similarly, for metformin, another diabetes treatment, affordability ranged between 0.6 and 10.8 days' wages for a 30-day supply of a 500mg tablet taken three times a day. In a smaller sample study of NCD medicines in six low- and middle-income countries, the affordability of combination therapy generic equivalents for coronary heart disease (aspirin, a statin, a beta-blocker, and an ACE inhibitor), varied between 1.5 days' wages in Sri Lanka to 48.8 days' wages in Malawi.[10]

Low levels of detection, diagnosis, and prescribing, often due to limited affordability for such care and treatment, leads many actors in the supply chain to believe the true demand for NCD medicines is low, when in fact there is a large latent unmet demand due to the high and increasing burden of NCDs. Accurate demand information is critical to ensure that manufacturing, procurement, and distribution stages of the supply chain are working in tandem to match the current need. In the private sector, lack of market information appears to influence poor availability of NCD treatments and diagnostics. A combination of suboptimal demand, including low levels of education of both patients and providers, may make it difficult for manufacturers and suppliers to understand the NCD commodities market dynamics. Likewise, demand for products may not increase, if retailers are not "pushing" the recommended combination of treatment methods and pricing products at a level that is affordable for individuals.

As a result, a demand and supply cycle emerges wherein manufacturers and retailers struggle to price affordably and increase market penetration for NCD medicines and diagnostics, which in turn fails to affect the existent low community sensitization/demand for the recommended options. Poor affordability as well as other dynamic, context-specific factors may lead to an increase in the number of Trade Related Aspects of Intellectual Property Rights (TRIPS)-plus and compulsory licensing cases, particularly within middle-income countries.[11]

Lack of Availability of Medicines

In general, availability of medicines to treat noncommunicable diseases also remains low. NCD medicines in low-income countries are available at a level that is only a quarter of that in high-income countries.[12] Availability of generic medicines (typically the less expensive option for treatment) to treat chronic diseases is significantly less than the availability of generics used to treat acute conditions in both public and private sectors, especially within low- and lower-middle-income countries.[13] It should be noted that while trends in availability exist across countries, significant variation has been cited in large multinational analyses conducted by the WHO and Health Action International (HAI).[14] In the 2006 WHO/HAI study of price, availability, and affordability of NCD medicines,[15] generic medicines were more commonly available in public sector facilities. In contrast, branded medicines were more commonly available in private sector facilities. Stock-outs in the public sector often meant that patients purchased more expensive generic and brand name medicines in the private sector or went without consistent treatment.

Availability of basic technologies and medicines for diabetes and cancer is especially poor in many low-income countries. In a study of six LMICs, insulin availability was reported to be particularly limited, with generic preparations rarely available.[16] Insulin use also requires consistent availability and affordability of syringes. The cost of diabetes care, specifically the cost of insulin and syringes, is outlined in table 2.2. In addition, insulin distribution requires cold chain specifications and utilizes supply chain configurations that are often distinct from those used for general NCD medicine supply chains. As a result, in order to ensure access to insulin, distribution, tendering, and government policies all require in-depth review, prior planning, and ongoing coordination.[17]

Country-specific labeling requirements and complex registration procedures, especially when the market size is small, sometimes lead to poor availability of

Table 2.2   Cost of diabetes care, International Insulin Foundation reports

Country	Insulin[a] (%)	Syringes[b] (%)	Testing[c] (%)	Consultation[d] (%)	Travel[e] (%)	Total $ per year	% of per capita income[f]
Mali (2004)	38	34	8	7	12	339.4	61
Mozambique (2003)	5	24	1	9	61	273.6	75
Nicaragua (2007)	0	73	0	0	27	74.4	7
Zambia (2003)	12	63	6	6	12	199.1	21
Vietnam (2008)	39	8	5	3	46	427.0	51

Source: Beran D and Yudkin J. Looking beyond the issue of access to insulin: What is needed for proper diabetes care in resource-poor settings. *Diabetes Research and Clinical Practice;* 2010; 88(3): 217–21.

Note: Percentages and amounts are of total costs for diabetes care per patient. Percentages may not add to 100 because of rounding.

[a] 1 vial per month.
[b] 1 per day.
[c] 1 blood glucose test per month.
[d] 1 per month.
[e] To 1 consultation per month.
[f] Per capita GDP.

products.[18] Products may not be registered or distributed at the national level due to these requirements and procedures. Opioids, used for palliative care and pain management of many noncommunicable diseases, particularly cancers, represent a specific category of medications with complicated registration procedures.[19]

Lack of Availability of Diagnostics and Medical Devices

Availability also remains limited for NCD diagnostics. In a recent study of global health diagnostics, RAND found significant need and benefits from scaling use of new diagnostic technologies. In LMICs, specific examples of increased diagnostic use exist; however, most of these diagnostics are utilized to detect communicable diseases such as malaria, tuberculosis, and HIV/AIDS.[20] Few efforts have been directed at integrating diagnostics for the priority NCDs. Over half of the countries in the world have no guidelines (or have only recommendations) for procurement and reimbursements for approved medical devices. With diabetes, some countries have worked to integrate diagnostic tools, most commonly the glucometer, into their national care provision. However, consistent availability of operational testing equipment, including glucometers, is a complex task to manage. Glucometers and testing strips tend to have a short market life requiring purchase of updated tools and strips. Often, countries will keep glucometers as long as they are operational, ordering new test strips when needed, but newer test strips are often incompatible with older diagnostic tools, rendering these tools inoperable.[21]

Results from the WHO Priority Medical Devices project revealed that at least one noncommunicable disease and associated medical device(s) was identified as a priority condition for each of the countries surveyed.[22] Despite this, many medical devices for NCDs remain unavailable and unaffordable to populations in low-income countries. For many NCDs, including chronic obstructive pulmonary disease, ischemic heart disease, diabetes, and cancer (malignant neoplasms), medical devices exist, but devices have poor availability, stemming in part from design that is often not suited for the context. Within each of these disease areas, opportunities exist for improving the adaptability, reliability, accuracy, and safety of medical devices as they function within low-income settings.

Without improved diagnosis, inappropriate treatment of individuals' symptoms and poor supply planning may continue to affect the global response to NCDs. Likewise, improved diagnosis without available treatments will deter individuals from seeking and potentially paying for diagnostic tools. Improving supply through concerted efforts in regard to both diagnosis and treatment is key to integrated management of NCDs.

Poor Implementation of National NCD Medicine Policies and Standard Treatment Guidelines

Many of the medicines included on the WHO essential medicines list for NCDs are off-patent, but adoption and coverage still remain abysmally low. One ongoing challenge is the development and use of coordinated national strategies to prevent, treat, and monitor noncommunicable diseases. In the 2010 WHO NCD country capacity assessment, of 22 countries with a high burden of NCDs, 77% had developed a national integrated NCD policy or action plan and 59% had actively implemented an NCD policy or plan.[23] Political will and allocation of resources, which are often limited, are needed to ensure implementation of national policy guidelines.

The width of treatments and diagnostics required for the integrated management of NCDs presents new challenges for patients, both in terms of affordability and adherence to complicated treatment regimes. In order to ensure care providers in both the public and private health sectors advise appropriate treatment, standard treatment guidelines need to be adopted at a national level and implemented countrywide. Drawing from the WHO's action plan for 2013–20, countries need to strengthen health services with the appropriate inclusion of information and resources for NCDs. As mentioned above, consistency of disease management is influenced by both individuals' ability to pay for treatments and also the availability of treatments at a subsidized price or free of cost. Appropriate disease management is also greatly affected by proper diagnosis and by patients' perception of the need for treatment.[24]

Many countries have NCD protocols or standard guidelines in place; however, few have successfully operationalized their guidelines.[25] 53% of countries surveyed (n=167) in the WHO's 2010 NCD country capacity survey, for example, have national guidelines for managing NCDs, but only 17% reported implementation of standard guidelines.[26] Further, the development of guidelines that are appropriate for available resources within low- and middle-income countries is often a challenge with NCDs. In certain instances, resource-constrained countries have obtained NCD guidelines, which are less applicable to their new context, directly from Western countries.[27]

Poor Quality and Lack of Supply Chain Integrity

Regulatory enforcement of the quality of NCD medicines and diagnostics is weak in many developing countries. The quality regulation function for NCD medicines rests primarily with national regulatory authorities, some of which lack the capacity or resources for appropriate quality enforcement across the supply chain. For some communicable diseases, the WHO prequalification program works with the national regulatory authorities and provides an international quality assessment process. No such systems currently exist for NCD medicines. Due to affordability constraints, patients often purchase less expensive, poorer-quality treatment alternatives for NCDs. Substantial resources are required to effectively prevent and track both substandard (poor-quality) medications and counterfeit (having copied branding and packaging) medications if introduced to a national supply system. Optimally designed supply chains will facilitate transparency and information collection; however, at present, the fragmentation across multiple entities does not allow such tracking and monitoring.

Lack of Leadership and Global Support Architecture

In the 2010 WHO NCD Country Capacity survey, most countries had focal points (i.e., health unit, branch, or department) responsible for managing NCDs within the Ministry of Health.[28] This indicates an acknowledgment of the importance of NCDs at the country level, but it is still not clear whether there is serious political commitment to pursue action. Further political will, financial commitment, and cross-sectoral harmonization of work will be needed to support a national strategy to integrate NCD medications and diagnostics into the public sector. (See box 2.1.)

Role of Supply Chains in Improving Access to NCD Treatment and Diagnostics

Supply chains play a pivotal role in improving access to NCD medicines. In this section we highlight the main functions of the supply chain, the different types of supply chains commonly used, and differences and similarities across different contexts.

Primary Functions of Supply Chains

Supply chains fulfill three primary functions: physical movement of goods and commodities, information gathering related to consumption and use, and

Box 2.1 PEPFAR Global Supply Chain Structure

Procurement	Storage	Distribution	Point of care
Procurement is financed by PEPFAR with working capital financing to maintain smooth procurement cycles	Three regional warehouses are set up and managed by private company RTT	Distribution is carried out in-country by government and in some cases, NGO entities	Training from PEPFAR for health clinics to provide appropriate diagnostic and laboratory services
Procurement is carried out by Partnership for Supply Chain Management (SCMS)	Buffer stock is held at regional warehouses to respond to unexpected fluctuations in demand and smooth ordering cycles	Distribution from regional warehouses is facilitated through ongoing coordination and support from SCMS on-ground partners	Ongoing coordinations between PEPFAR and local NGOs to provide mentorship and training
International transport to countries is coordinated through SCMS partners UPS and FEDEX	Buffer stock is currently financed by the United States government but other options are being explored	Programmatic support for the development and implementation of information systems through SCMS on-ground partners	NGO community work to improve patient education and adherence to treatments received from points of care

PEPFAR supply chain structure. SCMS = Supply Chain Management System.

The global response to the HIV/AIDS crisis provides a clear example of how the international community and national stakeholders can coordinate efforts to improve diagnosis of and care for a specific disease. Through large commitments of funds and political will in favor of scaling up HIV/AIDS programs, thorough planning and design of resource allocation to ensure an optimal supply was applied to each entity in the supply chain. The President's Emergency Plan for AIDS Relief (PEPFAR) represents a long-term, sizeable global commitment of funds that facilitated the development of a carefully designed global supply chain architecture for HIV/AIDS. A similar global support architecture for NCDs is currently lacking. Efficient allocation of funds, coordination of partnerships, and shared management of ongoing monitoring and forecasting for matching supply and demand are elements needed for NCDs at a global level. NCD action groups exist, but few create broad linkages across disease areas to improve and sustain supply chains for essential medicines and diagnostics.

financing, as the supply chain influences transaction costs in the market. The physical function of supply chains includes storage and distribution of the product from the point of production to the point of consumption, carried out while maintaining high quality and product integrity. Supply chains may be structured to seamlessly link a network of procurement, warehousing, and transportation capacities. Optimally structured supply chains create these linkages in such a way that quantities of commodities are delivered at the lowest possible cost with the highest level of product reach. An optimally designed supply chain may also play an integral role in information sharing and transparency among stakeholders. Effective information flows may improve supervision of substandard and counterfeit medicines entering a supply system. Information on trends in consumption and use of products are vital inputs into accurate forecasting and production planning for commodities. Likewise, technologically enhanced supply chains may reduce delays in payments between supply chain actors and reduce transaction costs in the system.

When physical architecture, information gathering, and financial management are well aligned and applied appropriately to contexts, supply chains improve the affordability, availability, and quality of diagnostics and medicines. The physical structure of a supply chain, when designed effectively, may include fewer divergent entities, thereby simplifying the overall structure and improving the efficiency of information flows. Improved information transparency may better enable appropriate stocking, with fewer stock-outs and supply imbalances. This would lead to consistent availability of medicines and diagnostics at points where patients seek them. Improved availability may in turn affect other behavioral health efforts to improve NCD treatment and management adherence. Another outcome is improved pricing and overall affordability of products. Fewer intermediaries often result in lower retail prices, due to a lower number of distribution markups at each tier. Decreased retail prices and higher availability lead to higher demand, since a larger portion of the need can now be met. This in turn leads to further decreases in prices due to economies of scale achieved by manufacturers and distributors. Improved affordability also reduces the financial burden placed on the patient purchasing medicines for chronic conditions more often and over a longer period of time.

Furthermore, less fragmentation in the market enables better monitoring of quality along the supply chain and adherence to standard treatment guidelines. It may also allow for improved tracking of the types of drugs procured and sold.

Supply Chains in Different Contexts

While most supply chains perform similar functions, characteristics of specific contexts (i.e., type of commodity, geographic qualities, flow of finances, cost of commodities, public vs. private treatment seeking) have necessitated a variety of forms, involving management by different actors. The primary supply systems include government or public sector supply chains, private sector supply chains and nongovernmental organization supply chains.[29] Given the heterogeneity of

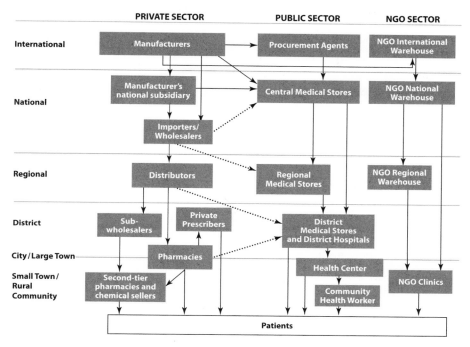

Fig. 2.2. Typical supply chain structures, by sector. Source: Yadav P, Tata H, and Babaley M. The world medicines situation 2011: storage and supply chain management. 3rd ed. World Health Organization, 2012.

supply chain structures, it is important to understand each sector's unique attributes, especially when designing an optimal architecture for the context of NCD medicines and diagnostics. (See fig. 2.2.)

Additionally, because procurement, distribution, and the overarching provision of pharmaceutical goods within a particular country are often disaggregated across the public sector, private sector, and NGO/donor groups, it is important to examine the opportunities for sustained integration and availability of a variety of NCD treatments and diagnostics. This requires further understanding of specific roles and responsibilities needed to ensure proper coordination, efficiency, and optimal market function.[30] Likewise, examination of transaction costs and opacity in the market due to excessive fragmentation will enable innovation around better retail pricing control for NCD treatments and diagnostics.

In most emerging markets, private sector supply chains for medicines include a network of importers, wholesalers, sub-wholesalers, pharmacies, and drug stores.

Pharmaceutical manufacturers sell products to national importers and whole-salers. In their current form, many private sector supply chains struggle to main-tain a distribution network with national reach. Additionally, many private sector supply chains include a large number of intermediaries between manufac-turers and patients and therefore struggle with excessive fragmentation and poor communication flow systems, resulting in limited coordination across actors in the distribution channel. Poor provision of credit is a challenge for different actors within the supply chain, especially retail pharmacies and smaller whole-salers who face high financing costs.[31] Eventually, high costs of financing are transferred to the patient in the form of higher prices.

Fragmentation of the wholesale market is commonly observed in most emerg-ing markets with large private sector markets for pharmaceuticals.[32] Due to the relative lack of distributors/wholesalers with nationwide coverage and reach, wholesalers often have to rely on sub-wholesalers or stockists, another layer in the supply chain, to reach retail outlets in remote regions.

In sub-Saharan Africa the predominant model for public sector distribution of medicines is to go through a Central Medical Store (CMS), which coordinates directly with regional or district stores. Transportation of goods is managed by a government/CMS-owned fleet. In addition to the CMS and regional or district stores, there are a number of primary and secondary distribution locations. These additional locations are present because of product- or program-specific supply chains set up by funding partners of the public sector.[33]

Distribution and delivery systems may also depend on the involvement of NGOs or faith-based organizations. Pharmaceutical delivery in this context is typically arranged according to the customer's own plan, courier services, drug supply or-ganization delivery services, or direct delivery services.[34] Variations in the distri-bution structures for this specific channel are considerable across countries.

Structural Similarities in Supply Chains

While the aforementioned heterogeneity exists among supply chain structures, certain similarities across supply approaches also occur. Most points of obtaining treatment (e.g., retail pharmacies, public clinics, or schools) are unable to keep large quantities of medicines in stock due to capital constraints. As a result, sup-plies are periodically moved from a district- or regional-level warehouse to health clinics in the public sector, while private wholesalers and distributors frequently move supplies from their storage facilities to their private sector clients. The num-ber of entities involved at different levels of the distribution system, the ownership and governance structure (publicly owned, privately owned, or public-private partnership), and the roles each entity plays may vary considerably by healthcare commodity and country context.[35] The basic movement of goods between points of use and points of purchase or in-country storage facilities remains relatively similar.

Recommendations for Improvement

A well-functioning supply chain is critical to countering the rising burden of NCDs. For sustainable access to NCD medicines, a range of changes need to be made to the global and local supply chain architecture. However, these changes can improve the effectiveness and efficiency of the supply chain only when there is an overall highly functional ecosystem for NCDs. The prerequisites of such an ecosystem include

- Healthcare workers trained and educated about NCDs
- Patient awareness of NCDs
- Availability of diagnostics
- Well-crafted healthcare financing policies that cover NCDs
- Better epidemiological data on NCDs to feed into planning and forecasting systems

Of these, the financing architecture for NCDs has the greatest influence on designing the optimal supply chain.

Global Financing for NCD Medicines

Although domestic country budgets and out-of-pocket expenditures remain the mainstay of financing for NCD medicines today, it is unrealistic to expect that a well-functioning supply chain for NCDs can be created without a change in the financing structure for NCDs. The poorest countries will need international support for their NCD programs, while middle-income countries will need political momentum to switch their health systems from out-of-pocket medicine purchasing to some form of pooling or insurance programs. In the short term, both types of countries would need to reprioritize domestic budgets to increase spending on NCDs in general and NCD medicines more specifically. In this chapter, we envision a model where NCD medicines in lower-middle- and middle-income countries continue to be financed through domestic budgets (medicines in public sector clinics), national or social health insurance programs (in public and private pharmacies), or private out-of-pocket expenditures (in private hospitals and pharmacies). In low-income countries, international support and domestic budget financing are envisioned to finance NCD medicines in the short term, with the objective of increasing domestic cofinancing gradually over time. This financing architecture and its associated assumptions provide the backdrop for many of the recommendations outlined in this paper.

Pooled Purchasing for NCD Medicines

Pooled procurement may provide one method for improving the affordability and availability of NCD medicines. While many pooled purchasing arrangements exist for essential medicines as a whole,[36] the Asthma Drug Facility is an example of a pooling arrangement aimed specifically at medicines for NCDs (e.g., asthma medications). Pooling procurement of healthcare commodities enables countries to negotiate for lower prices and provides suppliers with a forecast of demand from a larger community of purchasers rather than relying on individual tenders. Pooled purchasing also allows groups of buyers to obtain competitively low prices, especially for single-sourced products. In addition, it encourages buyers to communicate their needs well in advance, thereby potentially improving supply planning practices. In certain pooling arrangements, a revolving fund is used as an additional component to supplement timely reimbursement to suppliers until payment is received from buyers. Overall pooled purchasing reduces transaction costs for the suppliers because they do not have to transact with multiple smaller procurement entities.

In addition to its benefits, pooled purchasing also comes with a unique set of challenges. The presence of multiple actors in the pooling mechanism may introduce the same inefficiencies and delays in payment and shipments as with traditional individual tenders. Pooling, while improving procurement in the short term, may impact long-term market health, especially if the single buyer always prefers the least expensive source, creating reasons for other manufacturers to exit the product market. In the long run, this may cause more harm if it results in a supplier monopoly with one manufacturer controlling prices and supply. It is therefore important to consider pooling arrangements in relation to the context and community of participants.

For countries with relatively small NCD medicine needs, participating in pooled procurement arrangements may be of benefit. For larger markets with sizeable volumes of medicines, the benefits of a regional multi-country pool are less clear. In Mexico, a country with a large burden of NCDs, the government developed a new entity to negotiate pharmaceutical prices at the national level. The Coordinating Commission for Negotiating the Price of Medicines and other Health Inputs negotiates a procurement price for patented medicines, including many cancer medications, annually on behalf of all public institutions in Mexico.[37]

Differential Pricing for NCD Medicines

Pricing is usually seen as the key barrier influencing access to NCD medicines in emerging markets. For newer NCD medicines, particularly patented medicines, differential pricing is a sustainable way to provide access to NCD medicines to more people without compromising profits. Several examples exist within the field of NCD medicines. Novo Nordisk currently manages a differential pricing scheme for insulin in least-developed countries.[38] MSD created a differential pricing program for its diabetes medication Januvia.[39] GlaxoSmithKline provides differential pricing for a portfolio of 25 medicines, 15 of which are targeted at treatment of NCDs.[40] Merck Serono is piloting an intra-country differential pricing program for its diabetes medicines. AstraZeneca sells two of its breast cancer products, Arimidex and Nolvadex, at significantly reduced prices in low-income countries. Industry can play a central role in pursuing differential pricing for existing and new products. However, the long-term success of differential pricing requires cooperation from developing country governments, global agencies, NGOs, industry, and academe. In some cases formal partnerships may be established to ensure the success of differential pricing.[41] The NCD Alliance and other UN or multilateral agency task forces on NCDs should convene a platform that encourages continuing dialogue on issues that are preventing differential pricing from being used in a more scalable way. Supply chain factors that may be inhibiting the use of differential pricing are addressed through other recommendations in this chapter.

Comprehensive Picture of Need and Demand

Good demand forecasting is a prerequisite for building a highly functional supply chain for NCDs and even more broadly to increase access to NCD medicines. The NCD Alliance has stated that improved surveillance should be a primary objective of the NCD global agenda in their recommendations to the World Health Organization.[42] Governments and international agencies need demand forecasts for budgeting and resource allocation for NCDs, while the supply system needs the forecasts to plan logistics for NCD medicines. Frequently updated information on epidemiological needs, availability of financing (public or private), information on standard treatment guidelines, and user preferences for NCD medicines are essential to understanding demand more clearly. In addition to knowing aggregate demand at a national level, it is also critical to better understand where people seek treatment for NCDs (public, private, and NGO sectors), as this varies significantly across therapeutic areas and regions. Community-based surveys, in addition to hospital and clinic surveillance, will also improve the understanding of the global risk and burden of NCDs among populations not currently seeking care.

The information generation needs for NCD supply chains range from better synthesis of information that is currently available to gathering information that is not known and requires significant time and effort to be collected. We recommend that the following data be collected from existing sources to the extent possible, to feed into the supply chain planning processes:

- Epidemiological need for each disease category at national and possibly subnational levels
- Standard treatment guidelines used for different NCDs at national and subnational levels
- Market research on provider preferences for NCD medicines
- Market research on patient/caregiver patterns of treatment seeking for NCD medicines (public, private, and NGO sectors)
- Past consumption of various medicines
- Availability of funding for NCDs in each country from different sources

Building and operating a better supply chain is time consuming and will not occur overnight but through small incremental gains. In order to keep stakeholders committed to a path of progress that might be slow but needs to be maintained over time, it is critical to measure and report how improvements in the supply chain are leading to better access to NCD medicines. In addition to better supply chain planning, collecting the demand-side information listed above will also help populate performance metrics that track progress in increasing access to NCD medicines. Similarly, further mechanism analysis of supply and demand matching may prevent bottlenecks and inconsistencies in access within the supply chain. The International Federation of Pharmaceutical Manufacturers & Associations (IFPMA) may play a leadership role in this effort by commissioning annual market understanding studies completed by public-private partnerships (PPPs).

In the short term, ad hoc studies may help to develop a picture of need and demand. Further use of the Rapid Assessment Protocol first developed to monitor demand and supply for insulin may be appropriate for global monitoring of other

NCDs.[43] This protocol is currently being adapted to use diabetes as a "tracer" for other NCDs in communities in South America.[44] Similarly, the simple approach of developing a landscape paper on the demand and supply situation for each country and disease area, as used by the Global Access to Pain Relief Initiative for palliative care medicines, could be an immediate place to begin work (box 2.2). In the longer term, continued surveillance through the WHO STEPwise approach to surveillance, as well as other systematic methods for routine data collection, should be integrated into country surveillance and the routine Demographic and Health Surveys (in addition to current tracking within the Service Provision Assessment survey).[45]

Box 2.2 Global Access to Pain Relief Initiative: Country Report Methodology

Analysis of some basic data to describe the landscape of access to pain relief

Pain Treatment

Morphine equivalent is a metric to standardize doses of opioids by potency and allow the combination and comparison of different medicinal opioids. It is calculated as

Mor Eq = (1 × morphine) + (83.3 × fentanyl) + (5 × hydromorphone)
+ (1.33 × oxycodone) + (0.25 × pethidine) + (4 × methadone).

This equation is taken from the ratios of the defined daily dose (oral dosing for all except fentanyl, which is transdermal) as described by the WHO Collaborating Centre for Drug Statistics Methodology.[a] Because of methadone's widespread use as an opioid substitution therapy, nonmethadone morphine equivalent is also used in some instances and is calculated as

Nonmeth Mor Eq = (1 × morphine) + (83.3 × fentanyl)
+ (5 × hydromorphone) + (1.33 × oxycodone) + (0.25 × pethidine).

Opioid consumption data are taken from a dataset provided by the UN International Narcotics Control Board (INCB) with the release of their annual report for narcotics consumption.[b] For each drug, the average of available consumption data over the last three years (2008–2010) is used. Data are also published on the INCB website.[c]

Deaths in Pain

It is assumed that 80% of cancer deaths and 50% of HIV deaths require morphine and that the morphine required for each death in pain is 67.5 mg/day for 91.5 days.[d] The number of deaths due to cancer and HIV is estimated by applying the mortality rates from the 2008 update of the WHO 2004 cause of death dataset[e] to national population estimates for 2010 from the WHO.[f]

(continued)

Box 2.2 *(continued)*

Untreated Deaths in Pain
It is assumed that all of the morphine is used for deaths in pain due to cancer or HIV. The number of untreated deaths in pain is calculated by subtracting the number of deaths in pain that could be treated with the total morphine equivalent in the country from the total number of deaths in pain.

Source: www.gapri.org/methodology.

a WHO Collaborating Centre for Drug Statistics Methodology. ATC/DDD Index. 2011. www.whocc.no/atc_ddd_index/.
b UN International Narcotics Control Board. Consumption of principal narcotic drugs (1991–2010). 2012.
c UN International Narcotics Control Board. Narcotic drugs: Estimated world requirements for 2012—statistics for 2010 [E/INCB/2011/1]. 2011. www.incb.org/incb/en/narcotic-drugs-technical-report_2011.html; UN International Narcotics Control Board. Narcotic drugs: Estimated world requirements for 2011—statistics for 2009 [E/INCB/2010/2]. www.incb.org/incb/en/narcotic_drugs_2010.html; UN International Narcotics Control Board. Narcotic drugs: Estimated world requirements for 2010; Statistics for 2008 (E/INCB/2009/2). 2009. www.incb.org/pdf/technical-reports/narcotic-drugs/2009/Narcotic_drugs_publication_2009.pdf.
d Foley KM, Wagner JL, Joranson DE, and Gelband H. Pain control for people with cancer and AIDS. Disease control: Priorities in developing countries. 2nd ed. New York: Oxford University Press; 2006, pp. 981–94.
e World Health Organization. The global burden of disease: 2004 update. 2008. www.who.int/evidence/bod.
f Global Health Observatory estimates of population, 2010. 2010. http://apps.who.int/ghodata/.

Private Sector for Supply Chain Services

Currently, in many low-income countries the majority of medicines distribution is carried out by the government, through government-run Central Medical Stores and government-owned transport fleets. While some improvements have been made in government-run supply chains,[46] long-term sustainable improvements in the supply chain for NCD medicines will require increases in effectiveness and efficiency to levels that can be guaranteed through higher competition in the supply chain. It is worth clarifying that an increased role of the private sector in the medicine supply chain does not amount to privately provided healthcare or privately purchased medicines. Private wholesalers or private logistics companies can work in tandem with the government to ensure consistent availability of a range of medicines in government health clinics at the lowest cost. This requires strengthening the capacity of the government to contract supply chain services. While this capacity building cannot happen overnight, there is no avoiding it if a well-functioning supply chain that can deliver the highest value for money is the desired outcome. Partnership structures that include pri-

vate industry and country governments should be created to facilitate such capacity building.

High-Quality Pharmaceutical Wholesalers

Pharmaceutical wholesalers provide a vital connection between the manufacturer and the retail pharmacy / drug store. In many low- and middle-income
countries, the pharmaceutical wholesaling market is excessively fragmented,
leading to poor scale economies, poor coverage, and poor product traceability.
In order to have greater control over product flows, pharmaceutical companies
often select only one distributor/wholesaler as their distribution partner. While
this leads to higher control over quality, it may not always guarantee higher
market coverage and lower distribution markups. If pharmaceutical companies
were to work with three to four wholesalers/distributors in each country to enhance their distribution networks in both quality and reach, it would lead to a
healthy distribution market for NCD medicines in both the public and the private sectors.

   To avoid increases in transaction costs as a result of working with multiple
distributors, companies can develop pre-wholesalers in each region who could
then supply to three to four distributors in each country.[47] Such an approach
has been noted to both increase availability and decrease retail prices.[48]
Wholesaler strengthening should be accompanied by complementary initiatives
that would lead to smoother credit flows across various actors in the supply
chain.[49] To improve the quality and reach of pharmaceutical wholesalers in low-
income countries, global donors may coordinate training and other forms of
business strengthening with support from academic institutions and industry
organizations such as the International Federation of Pharmaceutical Wholesalers.
(See box 2.3.)

Accredited Healthcare Retail Networks

In addition to improving access to medicines and diagnostics through coordination and quality improvements at the wholesaling level, ensuring access at the
retail level is an equally important supply chain investment. One method for
ensuring retail availability of quality medicines, appropriate prescribing practices, and affordable pricing is through accredited healthcare retail networks.
Health-focused retail networks are part of the private sector, but they are often
accredited and maintain a certain quality standard regulated by the public sector.[50]
Accredited Drug Dispensing Outlets in Tanzania, CareShops in Ghana, and

---

Box 2.3 Case Study of Access to Medicines through Wholesalers

Procurement
Wholesalers typically maintain wide distribution networks directly to end-retailers or intermediate partnerships to end-retailers in remote and rural communities. Orders are collected on a regular basis using various ordering systems. Certain contexts ensure that technology, for example, Internet-based ordering systems, is used to reduce transaction costs and ensure up-to-date information. Orders are then pooled by wholesalers for purchase directly from manufacturers. Pooling enables wholesalers to negotiate lower prices for higher volumes of commodities.

Distribution
Wholesalers may manage a fleet of delivery vehicles. In South Africa, a fleet of 15 to 70 vehicles is tracked using a satellite system. Certain quality wholesalers offer 24-hour emergency service to large hospital groups. In China, 90% of pharmaceutical wholesalers utilize modern management systems such as e-order, warehouse management systems, and warehouse temperature and moisture monitoring systems.

Quality Assurance
Most national wholesalers are required to obtain licensure from the appropriate regulatory authorities. In South Africa, Good Wholesale Practice as well as Good Distribution Practice are followed by quality-assured wholesalers. Similarly, in China, the top ten wholesalers have International Organization for Standardization (i.e., ISO9000) and Good Storage Practices (GSP) certification.

Source: International Federation of Pharmaceutical Wholesalers.

Child and Family Wellness Shops in Kenya represent three similar models that provide extensive sales networks, with a specific emphasis on serving remote communities. Accredited healthcare retail outlets may be included in a national NCD strategy to increase access to and quality of available medicines and diagnostics. More specifically, franchise owners may be trained to diagnose, treat, and facilitate ongoing management of NCDs for individuals living in remote regions of countries. Linked with quality wholesalers, these two entities create a quality in-country supply system.

Global donors may support the initial development of an accredited healthcare retail network in low-income countries where such networks don't exist. Countries can then manage and enforce accreditation and quality standards through national regulatory bodies. The pharmaceutical industry may also play a role by providing preferential pricing to accredited networks.

Standard Treatment Protocols for NCDs

The creation of national guidelines and treatment protocols for NCDs will facilitate better adherence to recommended treatment options, enable better supply chain planning, and reduce irrational drug use. Poor adherence to guidelines makes demand for particular drugs difficult to track and predict. This in turn inhibits effective supply planning and may lead to stock-outs, supply imbalances, and overall, lower availability and higher total costs. Standard treatment guidelines (STGs) will enable healthcare workers at various stages in the healthcare system to make decisions about appropriate treatments for specific NCD clinical conditions. To ensure strong adherence to STGs, appropriate incentives need to be designed for prescribers and/or dispensers. If STGs are not enacted already, national governments should make their design and implementation a priority. The World Health Organization may provide technical leadership in this area.

Targeted Initiatives to Improve NCD Supply Chains

Numerous challenges and large-scale investment needs exist in the NCD supply chain. The work required to improve supply chains for all NCDs may appear overwhelming. The vast resources needed and the necessity for concerted efforts from multiple actors could lead to inaction. While a well-functioning NCD supply chain is not feasible without an across-disease focus, each NCD is different and may require a different set of tools, actions, and interventions in the supply chain. Improving NCD supply chains therefore warrants a pragmatic, context-focused, and adaptable approach. Selecting two or three disease areas with the highest burden in poor countries can lead to concerted action and serve as an entry point to build robust supply chains for NCDs. It is therefore essential to focus on specific diseases in different geographic areas and create a learning platform so that the knowledge gained from each therapeutic area and country/region can be expanded to other therapeutic areas and regions whenever possible. An umbrella partnership like the NCD Alliance may facilitate the selection and recommendation of appropriate disease areas for an initial focus. Disease areas and targeted interventions should be chosen using the best information available on the impact of lifestyle on disease status and challenges associated with access to medicines, diagnostics, and medical devices. Partners of the NCD Alliance, together with country governments and their development partners, could help implement the initial targeted programs.

For the selected few diseases and geographic areas, a coordinated demand and supply planning strategy can be created using processes similar to Sales and

Operations Planning, commonly used in the private sector supply chains. Such an approach will provide a well-coordinated operating plan to meet the estimated demand at the lowest cost using multiple suppliers for selected NCD areas. By first obtaining a complete picture of forecasted demand, a supply plan would be developed for a selected time horizon (e.g., month, quarter, and year). This plan would be developed through active discussion with multiple high-quality suppliers and other stakeholders in the supply chain. In addition, the IFPMA may help coordinate understanding of market conditions for NCDs through PPPs.

NCD Products Adapted for Developing Countries

Often, products must be adapted for the developing country context through modifications of packaging and appropriate administrative modes. For example, developing a resource-constrained version of defibrillators that are easy to operate and more affordable would help improve outcomes for patients with ischemic heart disease.[51] Manufacturers can play an important role in the development of appropriate technologies.

Interfirm cooperation in research and development through product development partnerships may be used to develop new NCD medicines, diagnostics, and preventative technologies.[52] NGOs such as PATH (Program for Appropriate Technology in Health) and other research institutions may assist with the appropriate adaptation of specific commodities for low- and middle-income countries and can help research modifications in packaging and more suitable modes of administration.

Better Regulatory Structures for NCD Medicines

Both health and the economy in developing countries would benefit from investments in their drug regulatory systems; however, bilateral and multilateral donor agencies have not strongly incorporated this into their current investment strategies.[53] NCDs provide a strong case for the value of investing in further strengthening of drug regulatory agencies' capacity in developing countries. Greater capacity for regulatory enforcement created with limited funding through international financing mechanisms would improve access to high-quality medicines and lower the risk of counterfeit products. In addition, these investments could help improve regulatory harmonization, along with reductions in the complexity of registration processes and specific labeling requirements, which sometimes prevent pharmaceutical manufacturers from registering certain NCD medicines in countries with small markets.

NOTES

1. World Health Organization. 2008–2013 action plan for the global strategy for the prevention and control of non-communicable diseases. World Health Assembly Document A61/8; 2008.

2. Geneau R, Stuckler D, Stachenko S, McKee M, Ebrahim S, Basu S, Chockalingham A, Mwatsama M, Jamal R, Alwan A and Beaglehole R. Raising the priority of preventing chronic diseases: a political process. *Lancet*; 2010; 376(9753): 1689–98.

3. World Bank. The growing danger of non-communicable diseases: Acting now to reverse course. Conference Edition. 2011. http://siteresources.worldbank.org/HEALTH NUTRITIONANDPOPULATION/Resources/Peer-Reviewed-Publications/WBDeep eningCrisis.pdf.

4. Maher D, Ford N, and Unwin N. Priorities for developing countries in the global response to non-communicable diseases. *Globalization and Health*; 2012; 8(14); Beaglehole R et al. Priority actions for the non-communicable disease crisis. *Lancet*; 2011; 377(9775): 1438–47.

5. World Health Organization. Essential medicines for non-communicable diseases (NCDs); 2011; www.who.int/medicines/areas/policy/access_noncommunicable /NCDbriefingdocument.pdf; NCD Alliance. Global monitoring framework and targets for NCDs; 2012; www.ncdalliance.org/targets.

6. NCD Alliance. Global monitoring framework and targets for NCDs; 2012; www.ncdalliance.org/targets.

7. Niëns L, Cameron A, Van de Poel E, Ewen M, Brouwer W, and Laing R. Quantifying the impoverishing effects of purchasing medicines: A cross-country comparison of the affordability of medicines in the developing world. *PLoS Medicine*; 2010; 7(8): e1000333. doi:10.1371/journal.pmed.1000333.

8. Lu Y, Hernandez P, Abegunde D, and Edejer T. The world medicines situation 2011: Medicines expenditures. 3rd ed. World Health Organization; 2011.

9. Gelders S, Ewen M, Noguchi N, and Laing R. Price, availability and affordability: An international comparison of chronic disease medicines. Background report prepared for the WHO Planning Meeting on the Global Initiative for Treatment of Chronic Diseases held in Cairo; 2006; www.who.int/medicines/publications /PriceAvailAffordability.pdf.

10. Mendis S, Fukino K, Cameron A, Laing R, Filipe A Jr, Khatib O, Leowski J, and Ewen M. The availability and affordability of selected essential medicines for chronic diseases in six low- and middle-income countries. *Bulletin of the World Health Organization*; 2007; 85(4): 279–88.

11. A compulsory license was provided to Natco Pharma Limited in India in early 2012 for an anti-cancer medicine, Sorafenib. www.ipindia.nic.in/ipoNew/compulsory _License_12032012.pdf; See also Francisco, M. Compulsory license bandwagon gains momentum. *Nature Biotechnology*; 2012; 30(9): 814. Glassman, A. A $400,000 drug and why it matters for global health. Center for Global Development Global

Health Policy Blog; 2012; www.cgdev.org/blog/400000-drug-and-why-it-matters -global-health.

12. World Health Organization. Global status report on noncommunicable diseases 2010; 2011; whqlibdoc.who.int/publications/2011/9789240686458_eng.pdf.

13. Cameron A, Roubos I, Ewen M, Mantel-Teeuwisse A, Leufkens H, and Laing R. Differences in the availability of medicines for chronic and acute conditions in the public and private sectors of developing countries. *Bulletin of the World Health Organization*; 2010; 89: 412–21.

14. Gelders S, Ewen M, Noguchi N, and Laing R. Price, availability and affordability: An international comparison of chronic disease medicines. Background report prepared for the WHO Planning Meeting on the Global Initiative for Treatment of Chronic Diseases held in Cairo; 2006; www.who.int/medicines/publications /PriceAvailAfordability.pdf.

15. Medicines included in this study were for asthma, diabetes, epilepsy, hypertension, and psychiatric disorders (14 drugs in total).

16. Mendis S, Fukino K, Cameron A, Laing R, Filipe A Jr, Khatib O, Leowski J, and Ewen M. The availability and affordability of selected essential medicines for chronic diseases in six low- and middle-income countries. *Bulletin of the World Health Organization*; 2007; 85(4): 279–88.

17. Beran D and Yudkin J. Looking beyond the issue of access to insulin: What is needed for proper diabetes care in resource-poor settings. *Diabetes Research and Clinical Practice*; 2010; 88(3): 217–21.

18. Mattke S, Haims M, Ayivi-Guedehoussou N, Gillen E, Hunter L, Klautzer L, and Mengistu T. Improving access to medicines for non-communicable diseases in the developing world. RAND Health; 2011; www.rand.org/pubs/occasional_papers /OP349.html.

19. Cherny N, Baselga J, de Conno F, and Radbruch L. Formulary availability and regulatory barriers to accessibility of opioids for cancer pain in Europe: A report from the ESMO/EAPC Opioid Policy Initiative. *Annals of Oncology*; 2010; 21(3): 615–26.

20. Burgess D et al. Estimating the global health impact of improved diagnostic tools for the developing world. RAND Health; 2007; www.rand.org/content/dam /rand/pubs/research_briefs/2007/RAND_RB9293.pdf.

21. Interview with David Beran, September 2012; Engineering world health. Projects that matter: Universal glucometer strips; 2011; http://ewh.tamu.edu/~ewh /sites/default/files/10-11%20EWH%20Projects%20that%20Matter.pdf.

22. World Health Organization. Medical devices—managing the mismatch: An outcome of the priority medical devices project. Geneva: WHO; 2010; http://whqlib doc.who.int/publications/2010/9789241564045_eng.pdf.

23. Alwan A, MacLean D, Riley L, Tursan d'Espaignet E, Mathers CD, Stevens GA, and Bettcher D. Monitoring and surveillance of chronic non-communicable diseases: Progress and capacity in high-burden countries. *Lancet*; 2010; 376(9755): 1861–68.

24. World Health Organization. Adherence to long-term therapies: Evidence for action. Non-communicable Diseases and Mental Health Department; 2003; http://whqlibdoc.who.int/publications/2003/9241545992.pdf.

25. Alwan A, MacLean D, Riley L, Tursan d'Espaignet E, Mathers CD, Stevens GA, and Bettcher D. Monitoring and surveillance of chronic non-communicable diseases: Progress and capacity in high-burden countries. *Lancet*; 2010; 376(9755): 1861–68.

26. World Health Organization. Global status report on noncommunicable diseases 2010; 2011; whqlibdoc.who.int/publications/2011/9789240686458_eng.pdf.

27. Mattke S, Haims M, Ayivi-Guedehoussou N, Gillen E, Hunter L, Klautzer L, and Mengistu T. Improving access to medicines for non-communicable diseases in the developing world. RAND Health; 2011; www.rand.org/pubs/occasional_papers/OP349.html.

28. World Health Organization. Global status report on noncommunicable diseases 2010; 2011; whqlibdoc.who.int/publications/2011/9789240686458_eng.pdf.

29. Yadav P, Tata H, and Babaley M. The world medicines situation 2011: Storage and supply chain management. 3rd ed. World Health Organization; 2012; http://apps.who.int/medicinedocs/documents/s20037en/s20037en.pdf.

30. Kraiselburd S and Yadav P. Supply chains and global health: An imperative for bringing operations management scholarship into action. *Production and Operations Management*; 2012; 22(2): 377–81.

31. Yadav P, Smith L, and Alphs S. Innovations in working capital for accredited drug shops. Arlington, VA: Technical Report MSH; 2012.

32. Yadav P and Smith L. Pharmaceutical company strategies and distribution systems in emerging markets. Chapter 12.18 in Elsevier encyclopedia of health economics; 2014; under review.

33. On average, only 52 percent of partners (i.e., donors) use CMS as their primary storage entity; Yadav P, Tata H, and Babaley M. The world medicines situation 2011: Storage and supply chain management. 3rd ed. World Health Organization; 2012; http://apps.who.int/medicinedocs/documents/s20037en/s20037en.pdf.

34. Banda M, Ombaka E, Logez S, and Everard M. Multi-country study of medicine supply and distribution activities of faith-based organizations in Sub-Saharan African countries; 2006; www.who.int/medicines/areas/access/EN_EPN study.pdf.

35. Yadav P, Tata H, and Babaley M. The world medicines situation 2011: Storage and supply chain management. 3rd ed. World Health Organization; 2012; http://apps.who.int/medicinedocs/documents/s20037en/s20037en.pdf.

36. Existing pooled procurement models include the following: United Nations Children's Fund, World Health Organization Procurement, Organisation of Eastern Caribbean States (formerly Eastern Caribbean Drug Service), Pan American Health Organization EPI Revolving Fund, Gulf Cooperation Council Group Purchasing Program, and Global Fund Voluntary Pooled Procurement Program.

37. Gómez-Dantés O, Wirtz V, Reich M, Terrazas P, and Ortiz M. A new entity for the negotiation of public procurement prices for patented medicines in Mexico. *Bulletin of the World Health Organization*; 2012; 90: 788–92.

38. Novo Nordisk. Differential Pricing; 2010; www.changingdiabetesaccess.com /contributions/differential_pricing.asp.

39. Harachand S. Hedging on the emerging: India-specific pricing bucks trend. Contract Pharma; 2008; www.contractpharma.com/issues/2008-07/view_india -report/hedging-on-the-emerging/.

40. Yadav P. Differential pricing for pharmaceuticals: Review of current knowledge, new findings and ideas for action; 2010; http://apps.who.int/medicinedocs/en /m/abstract/Js18390en/.

41. Goroff M and Reich M. Partnerships to provide care and medicine for chronic diseases: A model for emerging markets. *Health Affairs*; 2010; 29(12): 2206–13.

42. NCD Alliance. Global monitoring framework and targets for NCDs; 2012; www.ncdalliance.org/targets.

43. Beran D, Yudkin J, and de Courten M. Assessing health systems for type 1 diabetes in sub-Saharan Africa: Developing a "Rapid Assessment Protocol for Insulin Access." *British Medical Journal Health Services Research*; 2006; 6(17).

44. Interview with David Beran, September 2012.

45. World Health Organization. STEPwise approach to chronic disease risk factor surveillance (STEPS); 2012; www.who.int/chp/steps/riskfactor/en/index.html; Monitoring and Evaluation to Assess and Use Results Demographic and Health Surveys. The Service Provision Assessment (SPA) survey; 2012; www.measuredhs.com /What-We-Do/Survey-Types/SPA.cfm.

46. Vledder M, Friedman J, Sjoblom M, and Yadav P. The challenge of ensuring adequate stocks of essential drugs in rural health clinics: From evidence to policy. Washington, DC: World Bank, 2010; http://documents.worldbank.org/curated/en /2010/11/13720570/challenge-ensuring-adequate-stocks-essential-drugs-rural-health -clinics.

47. Mwenda J. Private regional distribution hubs for medicines in East Africa. Unpublished Master's thesis, Massachusetts Institute of Technology—Zaragoza International Logistics Program.

48. Interview with Iain Barton and Maeve Magner (RTT Health), August 2012.

49. Yadav P, Smith L, and Alphs S. Innovations in working capital for accredited drug shops. Arlington, VA: Technical Report MSH; 2012.

50. Bishai D, Shah NM, Walker DG, Brieger WR, and Peters D. Social franchising to improve quality and access in private health care in developing countries. *Harvard Health Policy Review*; 2008; 9(1): 184–97.

51. World Health Organization. Medical devices—managing the mismatch: An outcome of the priority medical devices project. Geneva: WHO; 2010; http://whqlib doc.who.int/publications/2010/9789241564045_eng.pdf.

52. Global Forum for Health Research. Health partnerships review; 2008; http:// announcementsfiles.cohred.org/gfhr_pub/assoc/s14813e/s14813e.pdf.

53. Riviere J et al. Ensuring safe foods and medical products through stronger regulatory systems abroad. Report brief. Institute of Medicine of the National Academies; 2012; www.iom.edu/~/media/Files/Report%20Files/2012/Ensuring-Safe-Foods -and-Medical-Products-Through-Stronger-Regulatory-Systems-Abroad/safefood meds_rb.pdf.

CHAPTER 3

Learning from the HIV/AIDS Experience to Improve NCD Interventions

Soeren Mattke

For only the second time in history, the United Nations General Assembly held a high-level meeting on a health issue, in September 2011.[1] This meeting addressed the growing burden of noncommunicable diseases in the developing world, which threatens to undo health gains made through better control of communicable diseases and economic growth.[2] The first such meeting, in 2001, was on the HIV/AIDS epidemic and galvanized a global response that achieved extraordinary progress in containing the epidemic.[3]

In spite of their different biology, HIV/AIDS and NCDs have much in common. For both, disease onset and progression can be delayed or avoided through preventive measures, but complete eradication is unlikely. Both are not curable with current treatment options and require lifelong treatment of the underlying disease and related complications. And both overwhelm under-resourced healthcare systems.

The goal of this chapter is to explore which lessons learned from the response to the HIV/AIDS epidemic can be applied to counter the rising burden of NCDs. In the first section, I argue that treatment has as critical a role as prevention but has received less attention in public discourse. In the second section, I propose that an effective response needs to rely on public-private partnerships and multisectoral collaboration. The third section applies lessons learned from the HIV/AIDS epidemic to improving NCD treatment, and the last section offers a summary and implications.

The chapter concentrates on diabetes, cardiovascular disease, and chronic respiratory conditions as a subset of NCDs that share similar considerations for access to treatment. (Cancer and mental health, the two other main groups of NCDs, require different treatment approaches.)

The Importance of Access to Treatment

Since health-related behaviors and lifestyle choices, such as diet, smoking, and exercise, play an important role in NCD causation, it would appear logical to focus on primary prevention strategies in combating NCDs. Surely, going to the root of the problems and addressing the underlying causes will allow the reduction of disease prevalence and progression in an effective and affordable manner. This focus on prevention is reflected in the World Health Organization "Best Buys" interventions, which emphasize preventive measures to reduce the burden of NCDs.[4] But it is important to keep in mind that those risk factors contribute to NCD causation but are not the sole causal agents, as is the case with infectious diseases. Genetic risk and aging, which preventive measures cannot influence, also contribute. Even people with healthy lifestyles can develop asthma, diabetes, and heart disease, and the prevalence of those diseases increases with age.

Nor is it true that prevention is always more cost effective than treatment of disease, because cost effectiveness depends on the "number needed to treat/prevent," which reflects how many people have to receive a given intervention to avoid, for example, one premature NCD death. Preventive interventions tend to require a much higher number of people, as they have to be applied to a large number of people who would never have developed the disease. Cohen et al. analyzed the cost effectiveness of various preventive and treatment approaches and showed that sweeping statements about the superiority of either are not justified.[5]

Finally, preventive measures tend to have a longer "time to effect," which captures the delay between the intervention and the change in outcomes. Rolling out prevention strategies today will not reduce NCD burdens for many years to come and certainly comes too late for the patients living with NCDs in low- to middle-income countries today.

Thus, reduction of NCD burden requires a balanced use of prevention strategies and treatment of manifest disease, as has been done in the successful fight against the HIV/AIDS epidemic.[6] The focus of the public discourse to date, however, has largely been on prevention. The UN Political Declaration, for example, calls out prevention as "the cornerstone of the global response to noncommunicable diseases" (paragraph 34) and discusses several preventive efforts in detail but devotes only one sentence to treatment (paragraph 44e).[7] But, while the focus of this chapter is on access to treatment, it should not be seen as underestimating the importance of prevention.

Several factors make access to treatment for NCDs easier than it was in the case of HIV/AIDS. First, it took several years to understand the biology of HIV/AIDS and develop potent drugs, whereas NCDs are well-researched conditions, for which drugs have long been available and for which an active drug development pipeline exists. Second, as we have shown in a recent report, patent protection for most of the first-line NCD drugs has expired and drugs are widely available as low-cost generics.[8] Third, there is no resistance formation with medications for NCDs, and thus drugs that are effective today will be effective tomorrow. In contrast, the HI virus continues to mutate, which leads to resistant strains and creates the need to continuously develop new drugs.[9]

Need for Public-Private Partnerships and Multisectoral Collaboration

At first glance, it should be relatively easy to provide access to NCD treatment. The diseases are well understood, safe and effective drugs are available and under development, and almost all first-line drugs are available as generics. In practice, however, fundamental obstacles remain.

The foremost obstacle is the magnitude of the challenge. The WHO estimates that around 34 million people in low- and middle-income countries lived with HIV in 2010.[10] To compare, there were an estimated 29 million *deaths* from NCDs in the same year, with prevalence being much higher.[11] This enormous burden of disease is affecting countries that at the same time hold the greatest burden of infectious disease, and the rapid increase of NCDs has left under-resourced health care systems to deal with a double burden.[12] India, for example, has the highest number of type 2 diabetics in the world[13] and, in 2008, faced 2.3 million deaths due to cardiovascular diseases.[14] At the same time, more than 2 million people die in India each year from malaria, pneumonia, and diarrhea.[15] Similarly, in Indonesia, communicable diseases account for 41% of years of life lost, while noncommunicable diseases account for 45% of years of life lost.[16]

This double burden is particularly straining for under-resourced health systems that have historically focused on care for acute conditions, such as infectious diseases, injuries, and maternity complications. Indeed, current models of care in developing countries tend to be vertically structured, with care delivery being encounter-based for acute conditions or disease-specific care (e.g., HIV/AIDS clinics). However, according to projections by the WHO, deaths attributable to communicable disease will approximately halve between 2004 and 2030 in low-income countries, while those attributable to more chronic NCDs will nearly double.[17] If current causal and demographic trends continue, there will be increasing gaps between services provided and actual service needs, the available versus the required health care workforce, and the actual versus the required health care plans and budgets.

At the same time, it is unlikely that, in dealing with NCDs, donor support can play a role similar to that seen in the case of HIV/AIDS. The HIV/AIDS epidemic triggered an unprecedented outpour of support that made it possible to stabilize the epidemic[18] and put approximately half of patients with an indication on antiretroviral treatment. To secure those gains in containing HIV/AIDS, continuous donor funding will be required for years to come, and budgetary pressure on donor governments will prevent them from making sizeable additional commitments.

Thus, a robust response to the NCD threat in the developing world will require public-private partnerships that bring together local resources, donor funding, and private sector contributions. Such partnerships have been successful at providing HIV/AIDS treatment.[19] In addition, the complexity of NCD causation and its widespread impact not just on health but also on economic development imply the need for a multisectoral response, as discussed in detail by Alleyne and Nishtar in chapter 5.[20]

Parallels to the HIV/AIDS Case: Where Can We Draw on Success Stories and Best Practices?

Timely Diagnosis

NCDs and HIV/AIDS share a long latency from exposure to disease manifestation and the fact that early disease stages have no or only nonspecific signs and symptoms. At the same time, outcomes are improved with early treatment. It is therefore critically important to educate patients and providers about risk factors and early symptoms so that affected patients can get diagnosed and referred to treatment. According to an analysis by the Global HIV Prevention Working

Group, countries that have been able to raise awareness, such as Brazil, Senegal, Thailand, and Uganda, share key elements of success, such as adequate and sustained financing, visible political support, evidence-based interventions (including local treatment access), use of mass media, anti-stigma measures, and multi-stakeholder collaboration.[21]

The impact of such outreach and awareness campaigns can be substantial. Ukraine, for example, instituted an opt-out model for HIV testing for pregnant women and achieved 90% coverage for measures to prevent mother-to-child transmission.[22] In South Africa, around 80% of young people are now aware of loveLife, a youth-friendly national educational program on HIV prevention and diagnosis, and its call center gets about 350,000 calls per month.[23] Overall, while population-based screening remains low, services for high-risk groups have been expanded significantly.[24]

Similar progress needs to be made in NCD detection. For example, about two thirds of diabetics in Kenya do not know they have the disease but present with seemingly unrelated complaints.[25] Awareness of having hypertension ranges between 35 and 46 percent in China, India, and low- and middle-income countries of Europe and Latin America.[26] A more recent systematic review showed that only between 10 and 50% of hypertensive patients knew about their condition.[27]

Improving early detection will require not only awareness campaigns but also better diagnostic tools:[28] A study conducted by the International Insulin Foundation found that only 6% and 25% of health centers in Mozambique and Zambia, respectively, could measure blood glucose levels.[29]

Some progress is being made. Kenya's National Diabetes Strategy, for example, focuses on awareness and empowerment of patients to promote early diagnoses and self-management.[30] Nokia and Arogya World, a U.S.-based nonprofit, collaborate on a diabetes prevention program in India that uses text messages. The program aims to raise awareness about diabetes and its prevention and hopes to reach one million consumers in rural and urban India over the next two years.[31] Microsoft funded a pilot project to allow remote screening for heart disease in rural Argentina.[32]

Referral to Appropriate Treatment

Much like HIV/AIDS, NCDs are not curable and require lifelong treatment, implying a need for referral to appropriate treatment after diagnosis. The global response to the HIV/AIDS epidemic created a robust infrastructure for care delivery. For example, the number of health facilities that provide antiretroviral therapy, which is regarded as a key indicator of health system capacity, expanded threefold, from 7,700 in 2007 to 22,400 at the end of 2010.[33] An important component of this success was the WHO's public-health approach to antiretroviral therapy.[34] WHO realized early on that developing countries lacked the resources to employ the rich-country model, with specialty care management, complex monitoring, and highly tailored treatment. Instead, the WHO introduced a simplified decision algorithm centered on the "four Ss"—when to: start drug treatment; substitute for toxicity; switch after treatment failure; and stop. Combined with standardized treatment protocols, this approach empowered lower-level healthcare workers to deliver HIV care. Task shifting from higher-level to less-trained healthcare workers, in particular to support and monitor treatment continuation, has been an essential element of sustaining treatment programs.

To solidify those gains, the UNAIDS Secretariat and WHO launched Treatment 2.0 in June 2010, which aims to improve the efficiency and impact of HIV treatment programs in resource-limited countries and ultimately ensure their long-term sustainability. Key components are optimized drug regimens, access to point-of-care diagnostic and monitoring tools for CD4 count and viral load, lower cost, delivery system redesign, and community involvement.[35]

Similar progress has yet to be made in NCD care. A recent study analyzing the WHO's World Health Surveys, conducted in 70 countries, found that only 32% and 37.5% of respondents with a chronic condition in low-income and lower-middle income countries, respectively, had access to treatment.[36] Only 20–40% of patients diagnosed with hypertension in China, India, and low- and middle-income countries of Europe and Latin America received any treatment.[37] Where access to treatment exists, providers might not be organized or trained to provide proper NCD care. Records, for example, are commonly kept by visit and do not allow tracking of patients with chronic disease over time.

Affordability of care remains a substantial obstacle, as according to the WHO's 2010 NCD country capacity survey, only 25–35% of low-income and lower-middle income countries have insurance schemes that cover NCD-related services and treatments.[38] While many, particularly the least developed countries, now have a donor-supported delivery infrastructure for HIV care, it has been designed for this narrow purpose and cannot be repurposed for NCD care without redesign.[39]

Given the magnitude of the challenge of addressing gaps in infrastructure and insurance coverage, most efforts to date have focused on the short-term goal of educating providers about NCD care, as they were commonly less familiar with this set of conditions. The e-diabetes program,[40] for instance, is a public-private partnership supported by Sanofi. It trains providers in francophone Africa through teleconferences on the diagnosis and treatment of diabetes using context-appropriate standards of care. Similarly, the Changing Diabetes in Children Program, a collaboration between the International Society for Pediatric and Adolescent Diabetes and Novo Nordisk, has developed training material for type 1 diabetes care for children in developing countries.[41] But more fundamental efforts exist, and Kruk, Nigenda, and Knaul have sketched an agenda regarding how to reconfigure primary care to improve NCD treatment. The government of Jamaica has created the National Health Fund, which is partly financed by a tax on tobacco products, to subsidize NCD care.[42] The Chinese Ministry of Health and the World Bank have jointly adopted a three-step approach, with the aim of placing NCDs at the top of the government's agenda.[43]

Access to Medicines

Access to medicines is a critical component of both HIV/AIDS and NCD treatment, and providing access to highly effective treatment has been a remarkable success story in combatting the HIV epidemic. The WHO and UNAIDS' (the United Nations Programme on HIV and AIDS) "3 by 5" initiative, launched on World AIDS Day in 2003, challenged governments, foundations, corporations, and the UN system to scale up access to antiretroviral therapy as quickly and effectively as possible, by setting a target of increasing antiretroviral therapy from 400,000 to 3 million people by the end of 2005. The initiative met its target in 2007, and by the end of 2010 the number of people receiving treatment in low- and middle-income countries had reached 6.65 million, implying 47% coverage of eligible patients.[44] According to calculations by UNAIDS, this success has averted 2.5 million deaths in low- and middle-income countries globally since 1995.

The success also highlights the power of committed public-private partnerships. Its key components were substantial donor commitments, such as the U.S. President's Emergency Plan for AIDS Relief and the Global Fund to Fight AIDS, Tuberculosis and Malaria, the Accelerating Access Initiative of the research-based pharmaceutical industry, procurement support by the WHO's AIDS Medicines and Diagnostics Service, and local government and nongovernmental partners.[45]

As mentioned earlier, providing similar access to NCD treatments should be possible. The diseases are well understood, and powerful medicines have been in use for a very long time. Almost all first-line drugs have lost their patent protection and can be procured as low-cost generics. Yet access to NCD medicines remains limited in the developing world. A recent study, for instance, showed that medicines for NCDs are even less available than those for acute conditions, particularly in low- and lower-middle-income countries and in the public sector.[46] Consistent with views expressed in other chapters in this volume, the authors attribute the low availability to factors such as regulatory burden, inadequate funding, lack of incentives for maintaining stocks, poor forecasting abilities, inefficient purchasing/distribution systems, and leakage of medicines for private resale. Markups along inefficient supply chains can render medicines that are cheap to produce unaffordable at the point of dispensing.

Resolving all these obstacles will be challenging, as it would require fundamental changes in governance and funding of healthcare systems in the developing world, neither of which seems likely in the short run. However, access to medicines can be improved by facilitating product registration through regulatory harmonization and increasing efficiency and safety of supply chains, as proposed by White-Guay and Smith and Yadav, respectively.[47] Mattke et al. have argued recently that pharmaceutical companies could expand the concept of branded generics. Currently, branding is used to assure patients of the authenticity of the product, but governments in developing countries might also be interested in a partner that can offer a full range of essential medicines and ensure reliable and secure management of the entire supply chain up to the dispensing point.[48] Novo Nordisk is currently piloting such a model for insulin in Kenya in partnership with local organizations and faith-based hospitals and clinics. Under this commercially sustainable model, the partners manage the entire supply chain and provide affordable access, even in remote parts of the country.[49] A similar model has been introduced by Novartis in India: Arogya Parivar is a commercially viable venture that delivers nearly 80 pharmaceutical, generic, and over-the-counter products, including vaccines, to poor and rural areas.[50]

Importance of Adherence

Near-perfect adherence is a critical component of effective antiretroviral therapy. Not only does adherence ensure reliable suppression of viral replication, but gaps in treatment increase the risk of resistance formation and therefore have public health implications. Recognizing this challenge, substantial efforts went into devising treatment protocols and tools to help patients comply with complex regimens that typically involve three different drugs for suppression of HIV replication plus other drugs to treat and prevent opportunistic infections. Bärnighausen et al. summarized the evidence for various types of interventions in a recent review.[51] They found that reminders, education, social support, improvement of nutritional status, and patient-centered care delivery all contributed to better adherence. The best evidence of effectiveness exists for text message reminders that have been evaluated in several trials.[52] Ware et al. undertook an interesting study by interviewing patients in Uganda, Tanzania, and Nigeria that had near-perfect treatment adherence and found that getting patients to see adherence as social responsibility and providing community support were key factors.[53]

An important innovation to facilitate treatment adherence was the introduction of so-called fixed dose combinations that combine three antiretroviral drugs into one pill. Studies show that such combination products improve adherence[54] and lead to better outcomes.[55]

Adherence is also an important component of managing NCDs. For example, studies have shown that adherence to statins and beta-blockers is positively associated with survival after myocardial infarction.[56] In patients with stable coronary artery disease, adherence to beta-blockers, statins, and angiotensin-converting enzyme inhibitors is correlated with a 10–40% relative decrease in risk for hospitalization and a 50–80% relative decrease in risk for mortality.[57] But low adherence rates are a universal problem. Studies conducted in countries as diverse as China, Gambia, and the Seychelles show that only 43%, 27%, and 26%, respectively, of patients with hypertension comply with their antihypertensive drug treatment regimens.[58]

As in the case of HIV/AIDS, low adherence can be caused by numerous interrelated factors, such as out-of-pocket cost, low levels of health literacy, the difficulty of treating asymptomatic diseases, depression, side effects of medications, and patients' lack of faith in the provider and treatment. The WHO groups these factors into five categories: socioeconomic and demographic, provider or health-system, patient, therapy, and condition related factors,[59] and Mattke et al. recently provided a summary of the evidence for those factors.[60]

Our review also showed that less research is performed on how to overcome lack of adherence for NCD drugs than for antiretroviral treatment. Cost to patients remains an important obstacle, as the retail price of low-cost generic drugs is inflated because of mark-ups along the supply chain and taxes and because NCD medicines are not as heavily subsidized as antiretrovirals.[61] Another important factor is the complexity of the drugs regimen.[62] Inspired by the success of fixed dose combinations for HIV/AIDS treatment, various "polypill" approaches have been proposed that combine multiple drugs like aspirin, statins, ACE-inhibitors, and metformin into one pill.[63] The polypill is a conceptually attractive approach, because diabetes and cardiovascular disease, as the most frequent NCDs, have risk factors in common. Proof-of-concept studies have been concluded, and confirmatory evidence for safety and efficacy is currently being generated, as my search of the website clinicaltrials.gov found seven ongoing trials.

Should those trials be successful, polypills could become the cornerstone of a secondary prevention strategy for patients at high risk for incident or recurrent cardiovascular events and achieve population-level benefits through risk reduction.[64] What should be kept in mind, however, is that polypills are a risk-reduction rather than a treatment approach, because they typically contain low doses of their active ingredients to minimize the risk of side effects. Thus, symptomatic patients may require a more tailored treatment regimen with higher doses. Further, the etiology of NCDs is considerably more complex than that of HIV/AIDS, and patients have different combinations of risk factors, symptoms, side effects, and manifest disease, which implies that we cannot expect success of the NCD polypills similar to what we have experienced with fixed dose combinations in HIV/AIDS treatment. But polypills can become an important first step to reduce NCD mortality in resource-poor settings, while we continue to strive for access to optimized treatment.

Summary and Implications

The global community currently faces a rising burden of NCDs that threatens to undo progress made in reducing morbidity and mortality and improving prosperity and economic growth. Initially regarded as a problem of the developed world, lifestyle changes and increased longevity mean that developing countries are more and more affected. At the same time, developing countries are ill-prepared to handle this challenge: their healthcare systems are resource constrained, focused on infectious diseases, maternal and child health, and injuries, and already challenged by dealing with communicable diseases, such as HIV/AIDS, malaria, and TB.

Prima facie, improving access to treatment for NCDs appears to be a more solvable problem than responding to the HIV/AIDS epidemic. The biology of these diseases is well understood, effective treatment approaches have long been established and, given that most first-line medicines have lost their patent protection, treatment costs per patient are low enough to make them affordable in all but the poorest settings. In contrast to communicable diseases, established treatments will not lose their efficacy due to resistance formation, and a robust pipeline will ensure that ever more effective drugs will come to market. Moreover, NCDs affect broad ranges of the population, implying that stigma and human rights issues are less of an obstacle.

But the sheer magnitude of the NCD burden and the complexity of this heterogeneous group of diseases create their own challenges. NCDs cause about 20 times the number of deaths as HIV/AIDS, and prevalence of NCDs continues to rise, whereas the HIV epidemic has been contained. Treating HIV/AIDS requires dealing with a defined, albeit complex, infectious agent, but NCDs are a mixed group of diseases caused by the interplay of genetic, environmental, and behavioral factors. And the global financial crisis means that a donor response of similar scale as the one to the HIV/AIDS epidemic is unlikely. Neither can resources be diverted from support of treatment for communicable diseases, lest the world risk a resurgence of those epidemics.

Creativity and innovation will be required to mount a robust response, and public-private partnerships will have to play a substantial role.[65] To successfully involve the pharmaceutical industry in such partnerships, two conditions must be met. First, the initiatives have to leverage core industry capabilities. Second, while they may require industry investment up front, they must be viable in the long run under local resource constraints and governance, since industry alone cannot sustain efforts of the magnitude required to respond to the NCD challenge. This chapter has identified three areas in which industry should invest:

1. Improvement of care delivery systems. The pharmaceutical industry should bring its considerable expertise to bear in order to help build NCD care capabilities and capacity. Developing countries commonly lack context-appropriate guidelines and training material for providers as well as patient education tools, and this chapter shows that companies can successfully partner with local stakeholders to fill this gap. Intensifying efforts, such as those described above, could improve access to quality providers as a key to better NCD treatment. Investing in improving the infrastructure for NCD care should also be in the best interest of the pharmaceutical industry, as it creates the preconditions for a sustainable market for medical products as countries grow wealthier.

2. Research on adherence solutions. Given the importance of long-term treatment adherence for NCD control, industry should invest in research and development of innovations to improve adherence. This

should encompass reminder systems and community support approaches, but also further research on polypills, if only as a bridge solution until tailored NCD treatment becomes feasible in resource-poor settings.

3. Development of sustainable business models to improve access to medicines. This chapter has pointed out several industry-supported concepts that offer safe, effective, and affordable care in low-income countries. Successful models have also been developed locally: a paradigm is India's Aravind Eye Care System, a not-for-profit organization that perfected an assembly-line approach to ophthalmologic care, combined with a sophisticated business model, to make cataract surgery affordable.[66] Industry should help to research and promulgate such innovative ideas.

Creativity and innovation alone, however, will not be sufficient to improve access to NCD treatment for the least developed countries and the poorest segments of the population in many developing countries, which will require transfer payments to afford care. The spread of health insurance schemes, such as in China or Rwanda, will help, and so will the introduction of commercially viable concepts that offer affordable care in countries without health insurance. Such innovative ideas can even become models for the developed world, where health care systems and finances are increasingly strained by the growing prevalence of chronic disease.

NOTES

1. Leaders Gather at UN Headquarters for a High-Level Meeting on Non-communicable Diseases (NCDs). 2011 High-level Meeting on Prevention and Control of Non-communicable Diseases, General Assembly, United Nations, New York, Sept 19–20, 2011. www.un.org/en/ga/ncdmeeting2011/.

2. Working Towards Wellness: Accelerating the prevention of chronic disease. 2007, World Economic Forum, www.weforum.org/pdf/Wellness/report.pdf.

3. Global HIV/AIDS Response: Epidemic update and health sector progress towards Universal Access. *Progress Report 2011*, World Health Organization. http://whqlibdoc.who.int/publications/2011/9789241502986_eng.pdf.

4. *From Burden to "Best Buys": Reducing the economic impact of non-communicable diseases in low- and middle-income countries*. 2011, World Health Organization. http://apps.who.int/medicinedocs/documents/s18804en/s18804en.pdf.

5. Cohen, J.T., P.J. Neumann, and M.C. Weinstein, Does preventive care save money? Health economics and the presidential candidates. *New England Journal of Medicine*, 2008. 358(7): pp. 661–3.

6. Mattke, S. and J. Chow, *Measuring Health System Progress in Reducing Mortality from Noncommunicable Diseases*. 2012, RAND Corporation: Santa Monica, CA.

7. Political Declaration of the High-level Meeting of the General Assembly on the Prevention and Control of Non-communicable Diseases. September 16, 2011, United Nations General Assembly.

8. Mattke, S., et al., Improving Access to Medicines for Non-Communicable Diseases in the Developing World. 2011, RAND Corporation: Santa Monica, CA.

9. Fauci, A.S. and G.K. Folkers, The world must build on three decades of scientific advances to enable a new generation to live free of HIV/AIDS. *Health Affairs*, 2012. 31(7): pp. 1529–36.

10. Global HIV/AIDS Response: Epidemic update and health sector progress towards Universal Access. *Progress Report 2011*, World Health Organization. http://whqlibdoc.who.int/publications/2011/9789241502986_eng.pdf.

11. Global Status Report on Noncommunicable Diseases 2010. April 2011, World Health Organization, pp. 1–8. www.who.int/nmh/publications/ncd_report_full_en.pdf.

12. Boutayeb, A. and S. Boutayeb, The burden of non communicable diseases in developing countries. *International Journal for Equity in Health*, 2005. 4(1): p. 2.

13. Diamond, J., Medicine: diabetes in India. *Nature*, 2011. 469(7331): pp. 478–9.

14. Global Burden of Disease: 2004 update. 2008, World Health Organization: Geneva.

15. Ibid.

16. Global Health Observatory: Data repository. http://apps.who.int/ghodata/.

17. Global Burden of Disease: 2004 update. 2008, World Health Organization: Geneva.

18. Dentzer, S., The unique saga of PEPFAR and its phenomenal potential. *Health Affairs*, 2012. 31(7): pp. 1378–9.

19. Sturchio, J.L. and G.M. Cohen, How PEPFAR's public-private partnerships achieved ambitious goals, from improving labs to strengthening supply chains. *Health Affairs*, 2012. 31(7): pp. 1450–8.

20. See chapter 5 of this book.

21. Bringing HIV Prevention to Scale: An urgent global priority. June 2007, Global HIV Prevention Working Group. www.globalhivprevention.org/pdfs/PWG -HIV_prevention_report_FINAL.pdf.

22. Towards Universal Access: Scaling up priority HIV/AIDS interventions in the health sector. *Progress Report*, February 2007, UNICEF, WHO, UNAIDS. www .who.int/hiv/mediacentre/universal_access_progress_report_en.pdf.

23. Pettifor, A.E., et al., Young people's sexual health in South Africa: HIV prevalence and sexual behaviors from a nationally representative household survey. *AIDS*, 2005. 19(14): pp. 1525–34.

24. Towards Universal Access: Scaling up priority HIV/AIDS interventions in the health sector, *Progress Report*, February 2007, UNICEF, WHO, UNAIDS. www.who .int/hiv/mediacentre/universal_access_progress_report_en.pdf.

25. Kenya National Diabetes Strategy 2010–2015. July 2010, World Diabetes Foundation, Republic of Kenya Ministry of Public Health and Sanitation. http://dia betes-communication.org/wordpress/wp-content/uploads/2012/09/Kenya-National -Diabetes-Strategy-2010-2015-Complete.pdf.

26. Adeyi, O., O. Smith, and S. Robles, Public Policy and the Challenges of Chronic Noncommunicable Diseases. 2007, International Bank for Reconstruction and Development / World Bank: Washington, DC.

27. Ibrahim, M.M. and A. Damasceno, Hypertension in developing countries. *Lancet*, 2012. 380(9841): pp. 611–9.

28. Mendis, S., et al., Barriers to management of cardiovascular risk in a low-resource setting using hypertension as an entry point. *Journal of Hypertension*, 2004. 22(1): pp. 59–64.

29. Beran, D., A. McCabe, and J.S. Yudkin, Access to medicines versus access to treatment: the case of type 1 diabetes. *Bulletin of the World Health Organization*, 2008. 86(8): pp. 648–9; Beran, D. and J.S. Yudkin, Diabetes care in sub-Saharan Africa. *Lancet*, 2006. 368(9548): pp. 1689–95; Beran, D., J.S. Yudkin, and M. de Courten, Access to care for patients with insulin-requiring diabetes in developing countries: case studies of Mozambique and Zambia. *Diabetes Care*, 2005. 28(9): pp. 2136–40.

30. Kenya National Diabetes Strategy 2010–2015. July 2010, World Diabetes Foundation, Republic of Kenya Ministry of Public Health and Sanitation. http://dia betes-communication.org/wordpress/wp-content/uploads/2012/09/Kenya-National -Diabetes-Strategy-2010-2015-Complete.pdf.

31. Gullo, C., Nokia to Launch Diabetes Program in India. *Mobi Health News*, Sep 21, 2011. http://mobihealthnews.com/13320/nokia-to-launch-diabetes-program-in-india/.

32. Mobile Diagnostic Kit Targets the "Last Mile" of Preventive Healthcare. External Research Digital Inclusion Program. Microsoft Corporation: 2007; http:// research.microsoft.com/en-us/collaboration/papers/buenosaires.pdf.

33. Global HIV/AIDS Response: Epidemic update and health sector progress towards Universal Access. *Progress Report 2011*, World Health Organization. http:// whqlibdoc.who.int/publications/2011/9789241502986_eng.pdf.

34. Gilks, C.F., et al., The WHO public-health approach to antiretroviral treatment against HIV in resource-limited settings. *Lancet*, 2006. 368(9534): pp. 505–10.

35. Oka, S. *Fact Sheet*. UNAIDS Geneva. http://data.unaids.org/pub/Outlook/2010 /20100713_fs_outlook_treatment_en.pdf.

36. Wagner, A.K., et al., Access to care and medicines, burden of health care expenditures, and risk protection: results from the World Health Survey. *Health Policy*, 2011. 100(2–3): pp. 151–8.

37. Adeyi, O., O. Smith, and S. Robles, Public Policy and the Challenges of Chronic Noncommunicable Diseases. 2007, International Bank for Reconstruction and Development / World Bank: Washington, DC.

38. Global Status Report on Noncommunicable Diseases 2010. 2011, World Health Organization: Geneva.

39. See chapter 4 of this book.

40. The e-Diabetes Programme: An innovative approach to improve diabetes care in French-speaking Africa, e-Diabetes. www.e-diabete.org/pdf/doss_presse_en .pdf.

41. Brink, S.J., et al., Diabetes in Children and Adolescents: Basic training manual for healthcare professionals in developing countries. January 2011, Changing Diabetes in Children. www.changingdiabetesaccess.com/FileAssets/ContentCast /35/CDiC%20Manual_UK_Jan_2011_001_LOW.pdf.

42. Non-communicable diseases in Jamaica: Moving from prescription to prevention. World Bank: Latin America and Caribbean (LAC) Region. http://sitere sources.worldbank.org/LACEXT/Resources/factsheet_eng2.pdf.

43. Toward a healthy and harmonious life in China: Stemming the rising tide of non-communicable diseases. 2011, World Bank: Human Development Unit, East Asia and Pacific Region. www.worldbank.org/content/dam/Worldbank/document /NCD_report_en.pdf.

44. Global HIV/AIDS Response: Epidemic update and health sector progress towards Universal Access. *Progress Report 2011*, World Health Organization. http:// whqlibdoc.who.int/publications/2011/9789241502986_eng.pdf.

45. Progress on global access to HIV antiretroviral therapy: A report on "3 by 5" and beyond. March 2006, World Health Organization: Geneva.

46. Cameron, A., et al., Differences in the availability of medicines for chronic and acute conditions in the public and private sectors of developing countries. *Bulletin of the World Health Organization*, 2011. 89(6): pp. 412–21.

47. See chapters 1 and 2 of this book.

48. Mattke, S., L. Klautzer, and T. Mengistu, Medicines as a Service: A new commercial model for big pharma in the postblockbuster world. *Occasional Paper*, Santa Monica, CA: RAND Corporation, 2012. www.rand.org/pubs/occasional_papers /OP381.

49. In Kenya, Novo Nordisk tests a new business model to improve access to insulin. Novo Nordisk Videos, April, 2012; Novo Nordisk A/S, 2012. http://video.novo nordisk.com/video/4872851/in-kenya-novo-nordisk-tests-a.

50. Improving Health in Rural India: Commercial innovation to address health needs at the bottom of the pyramid. Corporate Responsibility at Novartis: Sept 2012. www.novartis.com/cs/www.novartis.com-v4/downloads/corporate-responsibility /resources/publications/arogya-factsheet.pdf.

51. Bärnighausen, T., et al., Interventions to increase antiretroviral adherence in sub-Saharan Africa: a systematic review of evaluation studies. *Lancet Infectious Diseases*, 2011. 11(12): pp. 942–51.

52. Horvath T, Azman H, Kennedy GE, Rutherford GW. Mobile phone text messaging for promoting adherence to antiretroviral therapy in patients with HIV infec-

tion. Cochrane Database of Systematic Reviews 2012, Issue 3. Art. No.: CD009756. DOI: 10.1002/14651858.CD009756.

53. Ware, N.C., et al., Explaining adherence success in sub-Saharan Africa: an ethnographic study. *PLoS medicine*, 2009. 6(1): p. e11.

54. Jordan, J., Delea, T., Sherrill, B., Hagiwara, M., Richter, A., Tolson, J., Oster, G. Impact of fixed-dose combination zidovudine/lamivudine on adherence to antiretroviral therapy: a retrospective claims-based cohort study. Presented at the Sixth International Congress on Drug Therapy in HIV Infection, Glasgow, UK, November 17–21, 2002: pp. 17–21; Legorreta, A., et al., Adherence to combined Lamivudine + Zidovudine versus individual components: a community-based retrospective medicaid claims analysis. *AIDS Care*, 2005. 17(8): pp. 938–48.

55. Calmy, A., et al., Generic fixed-dose combination antiretroviral treatment in resource-poor settings: multicentric observational cohort. *AIDS*, 2006. 20(8): pp. 1163–9.

56. Rasmussen, J.N., A. Chong, and D.A. Alter, Relationship between adherence to evidence-based pharmacotherapy and long-term mortality after acute myocardial infarction. *JAMA*, 2007. 297(2): pp. 177–86.

57. Ho, P.M., et al., Medication nonadherence is associated with a broad range of adverse outcomes in patients with coronary artery disease. *American Heart Journal*, 2008. 155(4): pp. 772–9.

58. Graves, J.W., Management of difficult-to-control hypertension. *Mayo Clinic Proceedings*, 2000. 75(3): pp. 278–84; Guo, H., H. He, and J. Jiang, [Study on the compliance of antihypertensive drugs in patients with hypertension]. *Zhonghua liuxingbingxue zazhi*, 2001 Dec. 22(6): pp. 418–20, PMID: 11851054; van der Sande, M.A., et al., Blood pressure patterns and cardiovascular risk factors in rural and urban Gambian communities. *Journal of Human Hypertension*, 2000. 14(8): pp. 489–96.

59. Adherence to long-term therapies: Evidence for action. 2003, World Health Organization: Geneva.

60. Mattke, S., et al., Improving access to medicines for non-communicable diseases in the developing world. 2011, RAND Corporation: Santa Monica, CA.

61. Olcay, M. and R. Laing, Pharmaceutical tariffs: What is their effect on prices, protection of local industry and revenue generation? May 2005, World Health Organization: Geneva.

62. Adisa, R., M.B. Aluntundu, and T.O. Fakeye, Factors contributing to non adherence to oral hypoglycemic medication among ambulatory type 2 diabetes patients in southwestern Nigeria. *Pharmacy Practice*, 2009. 7(3): pp. 163–169.

63. Wald, N.J. and M.R. Law, A strategy to reduce cardiovascular disease by more than 80%. *BMJ*, 2003. 326(7404): p. 1419.

64. Smith, R., P. Corrigan, and C. Exeter, Countering non-communicable disease through innovation: Report of the Non-Communicable Disease Working Group 2012. 2012, Global Health Policy Summit. https://workspace.imperial.ac.uk/global-health-innovation/Public/GHPS_NCD_Report.pdf.

65. Sturchio, J.L. , More than money: the business contribution to global health. In The G8 Camp David Summit 2012: The Road to Recovery, J. Kirton and M. Koch, editors. London: Newsdesk Media Group and G8 Research Group, 2012, pp. 154–155. www.g8.utoronto.ca/newsdesk/campdavid/sturchio.html.

66. Aravind homepage. 2011; www.aravind.org/.

CHAPTER 4

Reconfiguring Primary Care for the Era of Chronic and Noncommunicable Diseases

Margaret E. Kruk, Gustavo Nigenda, and Felicia Marie Knaul

Chronic and noncommunicable diseases are a rapidly growing contributor to death and disability worldwide.[1] Conditions such as cardiovascular disease, diabetes, cancer, and chronic respiratory disease were responsible for 36 million of the 57 million deaths in the world in 2008 and were projected to cause 44 million deaths by 2010. While these diseases have traditionally been associated with affluent societies, 80% of the NCD deaths in 2008 occurred in low- and middle-income countries.[2] This change is due to population aging, urbanization, modified diet and activity levels, smoking, and substantially higher mortality among people with NCDs in poor countries.[3] Further, NCDs tend to strike younger people in low- and middle-income countries (LMICs), with one in three NCD deaths occurring in people under age sixty.[4] A graph from Brazil illustrates the massive epidemiologic shift in causes of death since 1930, with a dramatic decline in infectious and parasitic diseases and the rise of cardiovascular disease and cancer (fig. 4.1).

NCDs also cause pain and disability, with attendant loss of quality of life and productivity. Depression, which causes comparatively few deaths but much human suffering, is responsible for 14% of the global burden of disease, as measured by disability-adjusted life years, afflicting 121 million people worldwide, the majority

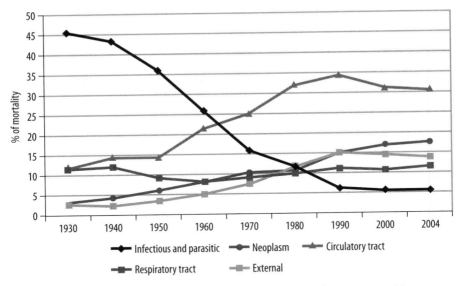

Fig. 4.1. Causes of death in Brazil, 1930–2004. Source: Pan American Health Organization / World Health Organization. Scaling up Primary Health Care Interventions for Chronic Disease Prevention and Control. 35th Annual International Conference of the Global Health Council. Washington, DC: PAHO/WHO; 2008. www.paho.org.

in low- and middle-income countries.[5] Untreated or poorly treated diabetes and hypertension result in painful complications and substantial lost income for families in highly affected countries such as India.[6] In many countries, NCDs disproportionately target the most vulnerable. Data from countries as disparate as Nepal, China, and India show that the greatest health and economic burden of NCDs accrues to poor and less-educated people within low- and middle-income countries, exacerbating social inequities.[7]

The staggering health and economic effects of NCDs in low- and middle-income countries are testimony to the dual failures of prevention and treatment. Recent estimates suggest that the total cost of cancer, for example, is 2–4% of global GDP and that investing in prevention and low-cost, highly effective care could save the world billions of dollars lost due to overly costly treatment, premature death and reduced productivity.[8] Tobacco alone is estimated to cost the world 3.6% of lost GDP each year.[9] Population-level efforts to promote healthier diets and physical activity and reduce tobacco consumption through policies, mass media campaigns, and tax instruments are at best fledgling, despite being potentially cost effective.[10] In an effort to draw attention to the NCD crisis and moti-vate progress, the UN held a High-level Meeting on Non-communicable Diseases in September 2011 that culminated in recommendations for population-level, multisectoral efforts to contain NCDs, emphasizing primary prevention.[11] Al-though this declaration was a step in the right direction, it is too early to assess the results of the political efforts to curb NCDs.

In low- and middle-income countries, secondary prevention—interventions to reduce disease progression and complications—is hindered by lack of aware-ness of risk factors among the population and health providers and low popula-tion coverage with screening and diagnostic services. More than 95% of cervical cancer deaths occur in LMICs, and the vast majority of breast cancer is detected in very advanced stages of the disease, when cure is impossible.[12] Recent studies show that only 20% of Tanzanians and 14% of Mozambicans with hypertension were aware of their disease.[13] Treatment rates, too, are low. Gakidou and colleagues showed that only 38% of men with diabetes in Thailand and 44% of men with diabetes in Mexico were treated, compared to 70% in the United States.[14] These figures are even lower in poorer countries.

The relative lack of attention to NCDs in LMICs, and the weakness of health systems in responding to the chronic nature of disease, is a function of the his-toric orientation of health systems toward responding solely to infectious dis-ease, malnutrition, and health conditions associated with pregnancy, childbirth, and diseases of the first years of life. The health systems of low- and middle-income countries continue to face the challenge of diseases associated with infections and other health conditions associated with poverty. This dual burden represents a polarized and protracted epidemiologic transition.[15] The diagnosis and care of NCDs requires a fundamentally different clinical approach, given the asymp-tomatic nature of early disease, chronicity, and frequent comorbidity. The thera-peutic aim in the treatment of NCDs is to minimize disease progression rather than to cure. In many LMICs, primary care providers are untrained and unequipped to screen asymptomatic patients, much less to provide life-long care to patients with NCDs. Further, health clinics are not organized to promote continuity of care. In low-income countries, healthcare funding is barely adequate to treat in-fectious disease, and much donor funding targets specific infectious and maternal/child health conditions, explicitly limiting use of funds for nontargeted conditions or general health system strengthening.[16]

Yet the damaging effects of noncommunicable diseases can be mitigated ef-fectively through a combination of population- and individual-level actions. Over the past 25 years mortality from cardiovascular disease (heart disease and stroke) has decreased dramatically in rich countries. In the United Kingdom, for example, mortality from coronary heart disease between 1981 and 2000 declined by 62% among men and 45% among women. Approximately 42% of this was due to clinical treatment and 58% to primary prevention or reduction in risk factors, mainly smoking, hypertension, and high cholesterol.[17] As this experience demonstrates, much of the opportunity in reducing the adverse health and economic impacts of NCDs such as coronary artery disease lies in prevention, early diagnosis, and treatment—the domain of primary care.

Primary care—defined here as first-contact care that promotes ease of access, care for a broad range of health needs, continuity, and the involvement of family and community—is perfectly positioned to be the main platform for the health system response to NCDs.[18] Primary care should address both primary prevention (e.g., smoking cessation advice, maintenance of healthy body weight) and be the main platform for clinical management of existing disease and prevention of sequelae, as well as provide palliation.[19] As table 4.1 shows, a great number of highly effective clinical interventions for NCDs can be provided by generalist health workers in a primary care setting.[20] Primary care should be seen as a component in an overall primary healthcare strategy that embraces the right to health and community participation and decision making.

But much has changed since the scope and organization of primary care were first defined at Alma Ata in 1978. Evolving disease epidemiology, including the HIV epidemic and rise in NCDs, uneven economic development, the rise of new communication technologies and social media, consumer demand for health system accountability, fragmentation of global health governance, and globalization of risk factors, have shifted the landscape of primary care in LMICs. As health needs and patient expectations have grown, so has the knowledge and capacity to meet the challenges. Yet as the state of NCD management illustrates, this knowledge has not been widely shared or implemented in settings that can benefit the most.

In this chapter, we discuss how primary care can be reconfigured to tackle the challenge of NCDs in resource-constrained settings. Our work builds on the emerging literature on the adaptation of primary care to the new realities of NCDs.[21] This reconfiguration will look different in various settings and will depend greatly on the existing health system. However, we suggest four universal elements that are essential to effective functioning of primary care in the NCD era: integration of services, innovation in service delivery, inclusion of communities, and information and communication for better care. We will review promising ap-

Table 4.1 Effective primary care interventions for NCDs

	Primary prevention	Diagnosis	Management and secondary prevention	Palliation
Cancer	Infant hepatitis B immunization (liver)[a] Adolescent HPV vaccination (cervical)[b] Decreased exposure to solar radiation (skin),[b] asbestos (lung)[b] Improved humid climate food storage (hepatocellular)[b]	Mammography (over age 50)[b] Fecal occult blood testing (colorectal) Clinical and pathological diagnosis (breast, skin)[c] Chest radiograph (lung)	Referral for breast, ovarian cancer surgery and radiation[c] Treatment of early-stage lesions (cervical)[a]	Home- and community-based care[b] Oral morphine therapy[b] Palliative radiation therapy (breast)[c]
Cardiovascular disease	Smoking cessation[a] Improved physical activity[a] Healthy diet,[a] specifically salt[a] and trans fat reduction[b] Safe alcohol use counseling[a]	Early diagnosis: blood pressure, cholesterol levels[b]	Multidrug therapy[a] Diuretic therapy[d]	Aspirin, atenolol, and streptokinase therapy[b] Benzathine penicillin therapy[b]
Chronic respiratory disease	Smoking cessation[b] Decreased indoor cookstove pollution[b]	Flow spirometry[b] Chest radiograph	Inhaled corticosteroids, beta-2 agonist treatment[b]	
Depression	Psychosocial intervention[e]	Adult opportunistic screening[f]	Antidepressant drug therapy[e] Brief psychotherapy[f] Suicide screening	

(continued)

Table 4.1 (continued)

	Primary prevention	Diagnosis	Management and secondary prevention	Palliation
Diabetes	Healthy diet,[a] specifically trans fat reduction[b] Improved physical activity[a] Weight management[b]	Glucose, hemoglobin A1C testing	Hypoglycemics[b] Annual vision exam[b] Retinopathy screening[d] Cardiovascular risk assessment Foot exams[b] Angiotensin converting enzyme inhibitor treatment[b]	

Notes: Cancers included here are breast,[b,c] cervical,[a] colorectal,[b] hepatocellular,[b] liver,[a] lung,[b] oral,[b] and skin.[b] Location of the relevant cancer is provided within parenthesis when restriction is indicated. Cardiovascular disease includes coronary artery disease, coronary heart disease,[b] hypertension, myocardial infarction, peripheral vascular disease, post-acute ischaemic heart disease,[d] and stroke.[b] Chronic respiratory disease includes asthma, emphysema, and obstructive pulmonary disease.[b] Depression includes all depressive disorders.[e,f] Diabetes includes both type 1 and type 2 diabetes.[a,b,d]

[a] WHO, World Economic Forum. From burden to "best buys": reducing the economic impact of non-communicable diseases in low- and middle-income countries, 2011. www.who.int/nmh/publications/best_buys_summary.pdf.

[b] WHO. Global status report on non-communicable diseases 2010. Geneva: World Health Organization; 2011.

[c] Yip CH, Anderson BO. The Breast Health Global Initiative: clinical practice guidelines for management of breast cancer in low- and middle-income countries. *Expert review of anticancer therapy.* Aug 2007;7(8):1095–1104.

[d] Ortegon M, Lim S, Chisholm D, Mendis S. Cost effectiveness of strategies to combat cardiovascular disease, diabetes, and tobacco use in sub-Saharan Africa and South East Asia: mathematical modelling study. *BMJ.* 2012;344:e607.

[e] WHO. mhGAP: scaling up care for mental, neurological, and substance use disorders. Geneva: World Health Organization; 2008.

[f] Beaglehole R, Epping-Jordan J, Patel V, et al. Improving the prevention and management of chronic disease in low-income and middle-income countries: a priority for primary health care. *Lancet.* 2008;372(9642):940–949.

proaches in low- and middle-income countries and conclude with implications for global and national policy makers.

Integration and Continuity of Care

Noncommunicable diseases share several features that have important implications for the organization of care. One, they are caused by many of the same risk factors. A high-fat diet, smoking, and being overweight, for example, are risks for heart disease, stroke, cancer, and type 2 diabetes. Two, comorbidity, or the occurrence of multiple noncommunicable diseases at the same time, is common. Three, some NCDs are in turn risk factors for others: diabetes for heart disease and stroke, for example. Four, they are chronic, lasting for many years and often decades. Five, while treatment can greatly reduce functional impairment, there is no cure for most NCDs. The goals of care are thus often not to cure but to enhance functional status, minimize symptoms, and prolong and enhance the quality of life, including pain palliation.[22] The chronicity of NCDs requires continuous monitoring and care as well as adherence to lifelong treatment. In this way, many of the noncommunicable diseases resemble chronic communicable diseases, such as HIV.[23]

As these examples make clear, the patient, not the disease, needs to be the focus of diagnosis, care, and treatment, and integration of care needs to move from the rhetoric of Alma Ata to reality.[24] Given the need for integrating prevention, diagnosis, treatment, and palliation across overlapping conditions, care by multidisciplinary teams has been proposed as a useful approach to NCD management.[25] This is challenging in low-income countries in particular, where health services are organized to address individual conditions or diseases, be it malaria, HIV, or obstructed labor. Donors stipulate separate funding streams for target conditions and make only limited investments in the health system as a whole. Health systems focused on episodic care thus fail patients with chronic conditions by neglecting to monitor disease progression and proactively work to prevent complications.

While in high-income countries integration of care implies removing boundaries between community, primary level, and specialist care, in low-income countries integration of care must begin with the reorganization of care delivery in primary care clinics, where today services are provided in silos.[26] For example, in most rural African clinics, patient records are organized by visit and not by patient, making follow-up and monitoring impossible. Patients are further segregated by disease: patients with HIV have separate registers, protocols, and often, different health workers from the rest of the clinic population. In such settings the very organization of health services is inimical to continuity of care.

Service integration in primary care in sub-Saharan Africa will require a dramatic shift in health policies and systems as well as in domestic and donor financing. Strengthening primary care platforms to meet the challenge of chronic as well as episodic care needs is part of a so-called diagonal approach that can strengthen the overall health system.[27] However, incremental steps may be feasible now. Rabkin and El-Sadr note that the massive expansion of HIV treatment in sub-Saharan Africa in the past decade has produced important lessons for NCD programming, given the similarities in the management of these conditions.[28] They point to successful experiences in establishing multidisciplinary care teams that include physicians, nurses, health educators, and other workers, introduction of patient-level medical records and appointment systems, and data systems that permit tracking of patient retention in treatment as models that can be used in managing NCDs.[29] Box 4.1 summarizes an experience from clinics in

---

Box 4.1 Adapting the HIV/AIDS Chronic Care Model to Diabetes and Hypertension in Cambodia

In 2002, two chronic disease clinics were established at provincial referral hospitals in Cambodia through a collaboration of the Cambodian Ministry of Health and Médecins Sans Frontières. These clinics sought to apply lessons learned in the management of HIV/AIDS as a chronic disease to diabetes and hypertension management. Medical personnel were trained in current treatment guidelines, and patients had individual records that were readily shared between services. Further, as per standard practice in the HIV clinic, financial barriers to access were assessed for each patient entering treatment.

All new patients followed an intake protocol adapted from established HIV/AIDS procedures. New patients were diagnosed and given a treatment plan in accordance with standard international protocols. Patient education and counseling were central, with substantial time spent from the first visit onward on adherence to drug regimens, healthy lifestyle improvements, and patient empowerment and responsibility. Psychosocial support in the form of peer groups was implemented to improve adherence and retention.

Two years after the clinics were established, 71% of the diabetes patients were in active follow-up, as were 90% of diabetes patients from the initial 3-month cohort. Participating patients reported high levels of satisfaction. The adoption of successful HIV/AIDS program components, especially psychosocial peer support groups and early patient education and counseling, in Cambodia led to high adherence rates after two years.

Box 4.2 Brazil's Family Health Teams Promote One-Stop, Integrated Care and Greater Health Equity

Brazil's Family Health Program is based on the Family Health Team, which includes doctors, nurses, dentists, and other health workers. By 2006, 27,000 Family Health Teams were active in nearly all of Brazil's 5,560 municipalities, each serving up to about 2,000 families or 10,000 people.

It has been estimated that annual resources for primary healthcare have increased in the past decade to about US$ 3.5 billion, with US$ 2 billion of that money devoted to the Family Health Program. Family Health Team professionals receive a salary as well as performance incentives to encourage effective and responsive care for their communities. The program follows the guidelines defined by the 2010 National Policy of Health Promotion to promote healthy lifestyles, healthy eating, and reduction of tobacco consumption, among other actions.

A recent evaluation by Mendonca and colleagues suggests that the large-scale implementation of the Brazilian Family Health Strategy in Belo Horizonte improved the quality of primary care services, especially in poor and vulnerable communities, where it reduced hospitalizations for primary care–sensitive conditions by 22% among women.

Cambodia that explicitly adapted an HIV chronic care model to the management of diabetes and hypertension.[30] While implemented in a referral hospital, most elements of this model can be replicated in a primary care setting.

Integration and continuity of care fare better in middle-income countries where primary care has been a policy objective for several decades and where health systems are better-funded and less dependent on outside donors. Team-based care, by teams composed of professionals such as physicians, nurses, rehabilitation specialists, social workers, and health educators, has been particularly effective at promoting ease of access, integration of services, and continuity in countries like Brazil, Mexico, and Costa Rica.[31] Box 4.2 summarizes the positive results of primary health teams in Brazil, which has made a huge investment in this model of care.[32] In both low- and high-income countries, team-based and integrated care require reforming the training curricula of physicians and nurses to accommodate their changed roles and promote collaboration.

Primary care in any setting also needs to be integrated with secondary, specialist care. In practice, such integration is rare. With the growth of urbanization in the region, integration of primary and secondary care will be made easier through proximity of communities to providers at all levels. However, this needs to be managed proactively—primarily through ensuring high-quality primary care that meets people's needs—to avoid high costs and overtreatment.

In Latin America, referral and counter-referral are haphazard due to segmentation of care systems and to perceived and real shortcomings in the quality of care at the primary level. In response, local institutions have been innovating to improve the coherence of referral. In Mexico, the National Institute of Cancer has set up a Network of State Cancer Centers throughout the country to provide primary care and refer patients who need specialized care to appropriate institutions.[33] State health units refer patients to Network institutions according to defined guidelines. Appropriate links with the rest of the health system will be needed to care for people with more severe disease and those who are not responding to treatment. Here primary care providers can play an important coordination role to ensure efficient and effective care.

Innovations in Service Delivery

Ensuring an Adequate Health Workforce

Scaling up prevention and care for chronic and noncommunicable diseases through primary care will require rethinking who provides services and how to ensure high quality of care. Shortages of physicians and nurses and urban-rural maldistribution are pervasive in both low- and many middle-income countries.[34] For example, while 45% of the world's population lives in rural areas, only 25% of doctors practice there.[35] This limits the potential of the traditional physician-centered care model in addressing NCDs.

Low- and middle-income countries struggling with physician shortages have led the world in health workforce innovations. One example is task shifting, or the devolution of care from higher-skilled health workers, typically physicians, to lower-skilled workers, such as nurses and clinical officers.[36]

Sub-Saharan African countries, including Mozambique, Malawi, and Tanzania, have gained extensive experience with developing new cadres of nonphysician clinicians (e.g., clinical officers, assistant medical officers, medical and surgical technicians) to lead in the care of infectious diseases, child and maternal health, and in some cases, general surgery. The results, as measured by clinical safety and effectiveness, rural retention of providers, and cost-effectiveness, have been encouraging, with quality of care being similar to doctors'.[37] One striking example of the potential of this strategy comes from Mozambique, where 90% of rural Caesarian sections are performed by nonphysician surgeons.[38] HIV programs have further extended the use of nonphysicians to the care of communicable chronic disease, with good results at low cost.[39]

There are comparatively fewer experiences in task shifting for NCDs in Africa, although several countries are embarking on nurse-led approaches.[40] Box 4.3 summarizes the experience with task shifting to nurses for the care of several NCDs in Cameroon.[41] However, task shifting should not be seen as an easy fix for weak health systems. It needs to be complemented by training more primary care doctors and reforming training to promote team-based care.[42] To ensure that new providers deliver high-quality care, they need supportive

---

Box 4.3 Nurse-led NCD Management Is Effective in Primary Care Facilities in Cameroon

Through the Cameroon Essential Non-communicable Diseases Health Intervention Project (CENHIP), an innovative public-private partnership, six pilot nurse-led primary health clinics were established in rural and urban Cameroon. Nurses implemented locally adapted algorithmic protocols, adhering to international guidelines for the care and management of patients with asthma, type 2 diabetes mellitus, epilepsy, and hypertension. Patients served by these pilot clinics include both direct CENHIP research staff–referred and local walk-in patients. Clinics were established in both private and public hospital locations with linkages to both the public and private health systems.

The protocols for the management of each NCD all included the following core elements: locally relevant algorithmic care of patients, disease management with essential medications, and patient education on disease and treatment rationale. Preclinic establishment and follow-up nurse trainings focused on the recognition and diagnosis of NCDs, management of care, improved record documentation, and referral procedures. Trainings were delivered through a mix of didactic lectures and hands-on practical supervised patient simulations. Some of the innovative approaches adopted in the program include

- Integration of services for NCD management
- Nurse-led primary care centers
- Point-of-care diagnostics
- Public-private partnership
- Patient-centered care and education

Select published health improvements include an average systolic and diastolic blood pressure drop of 11.7 mm Hg and 7.8 mm Hg ($p < 0.001$) and mean fasting capillary glucose level drop of 1.6 mmol/L ($p < 0.001$). Thus, nurse-led patient management supported by decision aids is a promising method of delivering care for NCDs.

national policies, stable financing, functioning supervision systems, and regulatory reforms.[43]

Country experiences show that nonphysician workers can successfully manage and monitor progress with cardiovascular disease. A study by Abegunde and colleagues found no statistical differences in the application of the WHO Cardiovascular Risk Management Package in primary care settings between nonphysicians and physicians.[44] The WHO recommends that properly trained health workers substitute for physicians in the care of patients with cardiovascular disease in settings where no physicians are available. These results were confirmed in rural and urban areas, including slums in northern India.[45]

Promoting Efficacious, Evidence-based Care

A critical concern in high- and low-income countries alike is the quality of NCD care. Attentive monitoring and proactive care is vital in ensuring effective secondary prevention of the sequelae of NCDs. Long-term drug therapy and frequent multimorbidity necessitate careful selection of medications and the ability to identify and manage adverse effects, which can be facilitated by clinical decision aids such as algorithms and protocols. As Wagner and colleagues noted in their influential 1996 paper *Organizing Care for Patients with Chronic Illnesses*, the use of explicit plans and protocols underpins provision of high-quality care for NCDs.[46] Decision aids and protocols can range from paper-based algorithms to computerized, patient-specific reminder systems. These can prompt clinicians about when to screen patients with diabetes for retinopathy and how to adjust the type and dose of antihypertensive medicines for patients with congestive heart failure.

Although NCD management guidelines exist in most countries, they are universally underused. Decision aids cannot be imposed top-down but need to be integrated into existing practices and supported by the broader health system to be viewed as useful by providers. For example, in Mexico, a three-session program of training, reflection, and problem solving using diabetes clinical guidelines among staff at primary care clinics, supported by visits by specialists to assist with difficult cases, increased good glycemic control from 28% to 39% of patients and improved achievement of other quality targets.[47] The use of protocols, with sufficient support from higher levels, was also central to the success of the programs from Cameroon and South Africa, discussed above.

In Latin America, there is an increasing awareness of the need to improve quality to achieve effective care for NCDs. Several governments, in partnership with professional associations, have designed clinical guidelines and implementation strategies to target high-risk or vulnerable populations. In Argentina, the government launched the Remediar+Redes program to strengthen the primary care model; it focused on a range of strategies to prevent and control CVD in uninsured populations.[48] The Institute of Clinical and Health Effectiveness, a nongovernmental organization managed by health professionals, has been monitoring the progress of the program to identify course corrections.

Expanding Diagnosis at the Point of Care

Expanding the detection and monitoring of NCDs implies a massive scale-up of screening and case finding, which in turn requires simple, accurate, and responsive diagnostics. Point-of-care testing, or testing that generates a diagnosis in real time, without need for a laboratory, is a particularly exciting approach in detecting asymptomatic disease early on, when treatment and/or secondary prevention has the greatest potential for impact.

Appropriate models will depend on the setting. One promising recent experience in scaling diagnostics comes from rural Uganda, where a five-day, multidisease diagnostic camp conducted a point-of-care screening campaign for HIV, TB, hypertension, and diabetes—using blood pressure examination and random capillary blood glucose testing.[49] The campaign reached 74% of the town's adult population and identified hypertension and diabetes in 48% and 3.5% of adults screened, respectively. Yet only half of those with disease obtained access to care at government clinics within three months.[50] Clearly, such campaigns are only as effective as the primary care system that can look after newly diagnosed patients.

These and other screening tests can also be provided at primary care clinics. One example of a cheap and relatively simple test that can save lives is visual inspection with acetic acid for cervical cancer and precancerous lesions. This test replaces the more complex Pap smear, which requires pathological examination in a laboratory; even a single test in a woman's life reduces the population risk of cervical cancer.[51] It has been shown to be highly sensitive in identifying disease and feasible to implement in primary care clinics in Sudan, Mozambique, Botswana, Peru, and China.[52] Box 4.4 shows how such screening can even be adapted to mobile outreach to improve access to care.[53]

Box 4.4 "See and Treat" Mobile Cervical Cancer Screening in Peru

The Peruvian League to Fight Against Cancer is a private nonprofit institution that has been using an innovative approach for early and effective diagnosis of cervical cancer among low-income women in Lima. Cervical cancer ranks as the most common cancer among women in Peru, and 7.5% of the general population of women are infected with human papilloma virus—the cause of cervical cancer. However, given the strained Peruvian health system, many women fail to get diagnosed or treated for this highly preventable and curable cancer.

The organization uses a "See and Treat" approach that dispenses with the need for a return visit. Each woman receives a visual inspection of the cervix with acetic acid, which allows healthcare providers to make onsite assessments and provide immediate recommendations to patients. Patients are all also offered breast, thyroid, and lymph node exams. All patients with a positive screen are referred to specialized care. Online medical records databases within the mobile detection unit track each patient.

The mobile units target remote and poor areas. To prepare a community for the screening, a social assistant spends time in the community to sensitize women to the importance of early diagnosis. The mobile units visit 4 communities each month and serve more than 5,000 women each year. Between 2009 and 2010, the league screened 37,774 women for cervical cancer.

The innovative experience of the Peruvian League exemplifies that innovative technologies, in concert with strong outreach, can dramatically scale up screening for cervical cancer in underserved areas.

Inclusion of Communities and Patients in Care

Reducing Financial Barriers to Care

In rich and poor countries alike, the burden of NCD risk factors and disease is highest among the most vulnerable members of society, disproportionately afflicting the poor and less-educated in cities and increasingly, in rural areas.[54] The poor have the worst access to health services and frequently suffer financial hardship from paying for care.[55] The success of primary care in tackling NCDs in low- and middle-income countries will thus hinge on inclusion of these populations in prevention and care.

While many governments in low-income countries have abolished user fees to promote access to maternal, child, and infectious disease services and witnessed increases in health care utilization by poor populations, few have done the same for NCDs.[56] This makes regular medical consultations and medicines unaffordable for a large proportion of the population with NCDs. For example, a monthly supply of insulin to treat diabetes cost 19.6 days of wages in Malawi and 25% of the minimum wage in Tanzania.[57] Health financing policies are needed to reduce barriers to access. Initial results from Cameroon suggest that reducing financial barriers by covering the cost of medicines every fourth month substantially improved retention of patients in hypertension and diabetes care, compared to a control group.[58]

To increase diagnosis and care seeking dramatically, NCDs should be included in the guaranteed benefit packages, and diagnosis and care of NCDs should be made free at the point of care.[59] In Costa Rica this approach has resulted in 98% of the population having coverage for primary care treatment of diabetes and hypertension.[60] While reducing user fees will cost governments money, expanding use of preventive interventions will reduce costly treatment of complications in the long term.[61] Some governments have experimented with cash transfers and incentives for vulnerable communities to improve lifestyle and healthcare utilization. In Mexico, through the Oportunidades poverty alleviation program, low-income families receive cash transfers contingent on positive health behaviors such as regular checkups. Evaluations demonstrated a measurable impact on body mass index and blood pressure as well as better self-reported health.[62]

Putting the Patient at the Center of Care

The keys to preventing and mitigating the health effects of NCDs lie in the hands of people with NCDs, not their doctors' or nurses'. Whether it is changing diet, quitting smoking, or adhering to medication for a lifetime, a motivated patient is the central partner in care.[63] The WHO's Innovative Care for Chronic Conditions framework further notes that patients need to be supported by families and communities, proposing that the triad of motivated patients, community partners, and health workers is the essential precondition for effective management of NCDs.[64] To achieve this, health systems need to treat patients as legitimate stakeholders—not just beneficiaries—of healthcare. This requires reinforcing the concept of citizenship in healthcare, that is, informing individuals about their right to receive information, to be able to use that information to change their lifestyle, and to be treated competently and with respect by health providers.

At the level of the primary care clinic, putting patients at the center of care means designing care systems to meet patient expectations and promote patient satisfaction.[65] This is partly captured in the WHO concept of responsiveness, or the ability of the health system to meet legitimate customer service expectations.[66]

Research in maternal health as well as in primary care and chronic diseases reveals that health system users have definite preferences about the organization, structure, and processes of health care.[67] For example, having a thorough physical exam and a physician who knew them well were far more important features of general practice visits in England than a short waiting time and flexibility in appointments.[68] Failing to recognize these preferences and to adjust service delivery accordingly reduces the utility of health care for individuals and hinders the effectiveness of the health system.

While important for all patients, taking account of patient preferences and expectations is especially crucial for people who have NCDs, which require ongoing contact with the health system and long-term adherence to therapy. Poor fit between expectations of the health system and services received may also discourage patients from taking an active role in self-management and participating in monitoring of health status—activities that require active collaboration and a trust-based partnership with health providers.[69]

Community Outreach to Promote Prevention and Enhance Care

The locus of most NCD risk factors is in the home and the community. It is here that individuals interact with social, cultural, physical, and economic structures that promote or impede positive health behaviors. It is therefore here that prevention and NCD management must be located. As the WHO notes in its Innovative Care for Chronic Conditions report, community leaders, nongovernmental organizations, and women's groups are well positioned to raise awareness about NCDs and the importance of healthy lifestyles.[70] Involving community leaders and groups in promoting prevention and diagnosis can reduce stigma and encourage patients to seek care.

Health systems are also increasingly reaching out to the community to support people with NCDs, using community health workers or peer outreach. Community health workers, non-health professionals who receive training in various aspects of NCD management, assist individuals and communities with prevention and lifestyle management, case finding of asymptomatic disease, and disease management. One of their main tasks is recruiting patients and families as allies in treatment. In addition, peers with the same disease—so-called expert patients— can be an important source for sharing experiences, best practices, failures, and emotional support for the frustrations and anxieties that accompany NCDs.[71]

A recent review on community health workers assisting with the management of chronic diseases in vulnerable communities in the United States showed that they were able to reduce blood pressure and promote adherence to medication in seven of eight randomized studies.[72] Some positive results on health behaviors and self-care were found in a similar review of community health workers and diabetes.[73]

There are fewer experiences with community health workers or peer support for people with chronic diseases in LMICs. Community health workers may be particularly useful in addressing diseases that are feared or stigmatized. In Mexico, efforts have been made to train community health workers in the identification and referral of women who have breast cancer. In Peru, the Dominican Republic, and Cuba, community health workers have been trained to identify individuals with mental diseases.[74]

There is also a growing body of experience with community health workers and HIV care. A recent review of programs in Brazil, Ethiopia, Malawi, Namibia, and Uganda found that community health workers with limited training can increase access to services and the quality of care for people with HIV, particularly in rural areas and vulnerable communities.[75] Box 4.5 summarizes the organization and results of a lay worker program to encourage better self-care for a range of NCDs in Shanghai.[76] The fairly low resource requirements of this program make it a suitable model for replication in poorer settings.

Finally, as noted in the discussion on task shifting, community health workers will not be effective in a vacuum. They need to be incorporated into the health team, supported by the health system, provided with ongoing training, and remunerated. Ideally, local communities should be involved from the beginning in planning and organizing their work.[77]

Information and Communication Technologies for Better Care

Chronic illness poses a variety of challenges for the patient, from changing habits and behaviors to adhering to daily medications to frequent interactions with the health system. All of these activities and more comprise self-management, the aim of which is to "minimize the impact of chronic disease on physical health status and functioning, and to enable people to cope with the psychological effects of the illness."[78] As noted above, these tasks require a motivated and supported patient but also a reliable and timely means of communicating health information between patients and providers.[79] Accurate information is also crucial to help patients navigate a sea of confusing information from media and the Internet. This area of healthcare has benefited from fruitful partnerships

---

Box 4.5 Lay Worker–led, Community-Based Training for Chronic Disease Control in Shanghai, China

The Shanghai Chronic Disease Self-Management Program adapted the Stanford University Chronic Disease Self-Management Program to improve self-management of a range of chronic diseases in five regions of Shanghai. One hundred thirty-one lay leaders, who themselves had chronic conditions, were trained to deliver seven two-hour sessions of a culturally adapted curriculum in pairs. Topics included exercise, symptom management, nutrition, fatigue and sleep management, use of community resources, adherence to medications, managing fear, anger, and depression, communication with health professionals, problem solving, and decision making.

Patients diagnosed with arthritis, chronic lung disease, diabetes, heart disease, hypertension, and/or stroke were placed into groups of ten to receive the intervention and compared to a control group without the intervention. In addition to education sessions, participants received a healthcare self-management book.

After a six-month follow-up period, patients in the treatment group (n=430) reported increased exercise, improved confidence in symptom and disease self-management, cognitive symptom management skills, and improved health status related to: overall self-rated health, health distress, fatigue, shortness of breath, pain, disability, and depression compared to the control group (n=349).

The authors noted that the program's success was in large part attributable to the participation of community governments and the integration of the program into community health services.

---

between industry (e.g., mobile phone and pharmaceutical companies) and the health sector.

Improving Lifestyles, Health Outcomes, and Retention in Care Using Mobile Phones

Mobile telephones are a near-ubiquitous aspect of daily life throughout the globe: in 2006 there were an estimated 3.3 billion mobile phones, or one for every other person in the world at that time. While over 90% of people in rich countries own a mobile phone, people in poor countries are fast catching up, with penetration of 33% in rural areas and 90% in many urban areas.[80]

It is therefore not surprising that mobile technology is increasingly being harnessed for healthcare. A recent WHO survey showed that 60% of high-income countries and 30% of low-income countries reported using text message or other mobile applications in the health sector (m-health).[81] The most common m-health applications include health promotion (e.g., reminders on smoking cessation or exercise), treatment adherence (e.g., medication reminders), appointment reminders, provider-patient communication (e.g., test results, monitoring), and patient-to-provider communication (e.g., glucose results, weight, management questions). M-health is one component of the broader e-health revolution that includes electronic medical records, web-based patient records, health literacy, social networking, and other informatics approaches.[82]

M-health is particularly relevant to LMICs, because computer ownership and Internet access lag behind mobile phone use in these countries. M-health also has the potential to bridge long distances between patients with NCDs and their primary care clinics. The global growth in m-health vastly outpaces its evaluation, but some of the early findings are encouraging.

A 2010 review of text messaging for health identified 12 quasi-random or random studies, all but one from high-income countries. Eight out of nine of the highest-quality studies identified positive effects on behavior change.[83] Other reviews also suggest positive effects on health behaviors[84] and patient attendance for medical appointments.[85] In a meta-analysis of mobile phone technology in diabetes management, Liang and colleagues found statistically significant declines in glycosylated hemoglobin—a marker of effective glucose control—in the pooled intervention group.[86]

A 2009 Cochrane review of texting and smoking cessation found short-term improvements that were generally not sustained over the longer run.[87] However, a more recent large randomized study of 5,800 Britons, half of whom received motivational messages and smoking cessation behavioral support and half of whom received unrelated text messages, found double the levels of abstinence from cigarettes at 6 months (10.9% versus 4.9%) in the motivated group—a result that was biochemically verified.[88]

There are no studies of comparable quality on m-health for chronic disease control in LMICs. The best-researched area of m-health in resource constrained settings is its use in the management of HIV. A recent Cochrane review found that weekly text messages, as opposed to standard care, enhanced adherence to medication and noted that one trial showed positive effects on viral load suppression.[89] The example in box 4.6 highlights a recent experience with diabetes management support using mobile phones in Honduras.[90]

The few evaluations of LMICs that exist are plagued by small samples, lack of comparison groups, and very short time frames for analysis. The last factor is particularly troubling in the context of chronic diseases, where long-term maintenance

---

Box 4.6 M-health for Diabetes Self-Management in Honduras

A recent primary care study found that 78.2% of the outpatient population suffering from common chronic diseases in Honduras reported having their own mobile phones, with 83.8% reporting having access to either a mobile or landline phone. Leveraging this abundant mobile phone usage, investigators piloted (n=94) a cloud-computing communications health promotion model built to improve diabetes self-management. Over a six-week period, patients received weekly interactive voice response calls delivering recorded personal diabetes management education messages. Calls also recorded patients' real-time personal health information and behaviors.

After a completed patient call, relevant information was emailed to the provider and a voice message was sent to the designated informal caregiver, if one was designated. At six weeks, HbA1c concentrations significantly improved, from 10.0% at baseline to 8.9% at completion ($p < 0.01$), with individuals who completed more than half the calls showing a significantly greater decrease ($p = 0.04$) in levels than those who completed less than half their calls. Participants reported that over the course of the study, they had improved their blood glucose control, diet, treatment adherence, and preventive foot care. This intervention met the needs of high-risk patients, with greater levels of call completion observed in patients with longer travel times to the nearest health center, raised blood pressure, and heightened diabetes distress levels.

This innovative pilot program, although brief, illustrates how existing technology and social behaviors can be leveraged to improve patient management of a chronic disease such as diabetes.

---

is essential for secondary prevention. The research agenda for m-health needs to also include economic evaluations to justify investments in this versus other modalities, as well as factors such as cultural context, sustainability, and integration with the health system.[91]

Evaluation and Accountability

There is a striking dearth of evidence for the effectiveness and equity of innovative approaches to tackling NCDs in primary care. Few of the many approaches being implemented today are accompanied by robust evaluation. Evaluation plays three important roles: it is essential for learning what works across settings, making necessary course corrections in existing programs, and promoting accountability to consumers and funders.

Evaluation of health system interventions is by no means straightforward. Assessing the health impact of a new NCD policy or clinical approach is complicated by the presence of multiple intervention components, difficulty in attributing health effects to program interventions, long time frames to see clinically meaningful change, the presence of confounders such as other programs and policies aimed at the same condition, and secular change.

Some of these factors, particularly the role of confounders and secular change, can be addressed by including control groups to permit comparison of changes between treated and untreated individuals or groups. While assigning people or areas to no treatment can be politically challenging when the programs to be evaluated are delivered or funded by the government, researchers can take advantage of gradual implementation of the program to make comparisons. Experience in Mexico shows that controlled evaluation can be done and can be tremendously instructive.

Box 4.7 summarizes Mexico's investment in evaluating its health insurance reforms and highlights how results of the evaluation guided health system change and promoted government accountability.[92] A welcome side benefit of Mexico's evaluation was the strengthening of data collection in facilities and communities that established a platform for an improved health information system. Where randomized evaluations are not possible, novel approaches such as quasi-random step-wedge designs, single and multiple time series, modeling-based analysis, and others should be considered.

In addition to having a rigorous research design, any evaluation of chronic disease initiatives needs to account for the role of context and fidelity of implementation in enhancing or hindering the effectiveness of programs. For example, factors such as local disease prevalence, capacity of local health managers, availability of drugs, skills of health workers, and other health system characteristics dramatically influenced the effectiveness of an international primary care initiative to improve care for sick children in different countries.[93]

Issues of context and quality of implementation lie in the domain of implementation science. Implementation science is the study of methods to promote uptake of evidence-based interventions at scale in real-world settings.[94] Its aim is to identify drivers of and barriers to implementation, recognizing that these may be due to local context, including factors such as disease prevalence, community preferences, utilization patterns, infrastructure, presence of other programs, degree of political commitment, capacity of district health managers, and mix and motivation of health workers.[95] It is essential to understand these factors if chronic disease initiatives are to be sustained successfully.

Box 4.7 Mexico's Health System Reform Evaluation Strategy

In 2003, Mexico launched its Social Health Protection Program (SHPP), aimed at allocating financial resources to provide healthcare to 50 million previously uninsured Mexicans. The program defined a package of 284 primary and secondary care interventions and funded both health promotion and prevention. One of the major features of SHPP was its built-in evaluation design. The SHPP design itself was heavily based on a body of evidence from health accounts and economic evaluation exercises.[a] Before the program was implemented, the Ministry of Health created, in 2001, a General Direction of Performance Evaluation to commission mandatory external evaluations of all priority programs, including SHPP. The regulations stipulated three types of evaluations: (1) managerial processes, (2) economic, and (3) health status impact.

Between 2004 and 2012, the ministry commissioned several managerial processes and economic evaluations and requested an impact evaluation in 2005. This evaluation was carried out by the National Institute of Public Health and the Harvard School of Public Health. A quasi-experimental design was used to assess (1) change in health status, (2) financial protection, and (3) responsiveness. The evaluation found signs of improvement, particularly in financial protection indicators, over the first three years of the SHPP. However, the authors concluded that the time was too short to allow for the observation of major changes.

In 2009, a third round of data was collected using the same population sample frame. This population sample was designed to carry out the original 2005–6 evaluation, and it was used in 2009 to assess the behavior of outcome variables. No changes were identified in 2009, compared to the original data set. Important improvements in household financial protection and responsiveness were found, showing the success of SHPP in reducing the gaps between the insured and the previously uninsured populations.

Managerial evaluations were also carried out in 2006, 2007, 2009 and 2011, and they show flaws in the purchasing and distribution of medicines, the contracting of health personnel, the allocation of financial resources, and the interaction between federal and state SHPP units. Some of the recommendations of these evaluations have been followed over the years by SHPP central coordinators to adjust processes.[b] Mexico's experience demonstrates how process and impact evaluations are crucial to the success of health policies.

---

[a] Frenk J, Knaul F, Gómez-Dantés O, et al. Financiamiento justo y protección social universal: la reforma estructural del sistema de salud de México. 1st ed. Mexico: Secretaría de Salud;2004.

[b] Sistema de Protección Social en Salud. Evaluación de procesos. 2006. Mexico: Secretaría de Salud;2007; González-Block MA, Nigenda G, et al. Evaluación del Sistema de Protección Social en Salud, 2007. Resumen Ejecutivo. Mexico: Instituto Nacional de Salud Pública;2008; Nigenda G, González G, Aracena B, et al. Evaluación del Sistema de Protección Social en Salud, 2009. Resumen ejecutivo. Mexico: Instituto Nacional de Salud Pública;2010; Nigenda G, López-Ridaura R, González-Robledo LM, et al. Evaluación externa del Sistema de Protección Social en Salud 2011. Resumen ejecutivo. Mexico: National Institute of Public Health;2012. www.dged.salud.gob.mx/contenidos/evaluacion_programas/descargas/spss/externas/EXT11_SPSS_SE.pdf.

Conclusion

While primary prevention of NCDs is largely the task of public health actions and policies across multiple sectors, mitigating the health and economic consequences of the burgeoning epidemic of chronic disease in low- and middle-income countries requires strong and resilient health systems. Primary care, care that is closest to the patient and the community and focused on the whole patient rather than a single organ or disease, has a starring role in the fight against NCDs. Primary care can prevent complications, slow pathogenesis, and enable people with chronic disease to live a full life.

Yet while considerable attention has been paid to strengthening health systems and primary care in LMICs to address traditional health threats in developing regions, principally infectious diseases and maternal and child health, there is less emphasis on preparing those systems to respond to NCDs. This is the case despite the fact that NCDs are today the most common cause of death in most LMICs. Even in Africa, which is still struggling with infectious and perinatal conditions, more people will die of an NCD than any other cause by 2030.[96]

In this chapter, we have built on earlier work by Frenk, Beaglehole, and others who propose rethinking the role and structure of primary care in this new age.[97] Our recommendations suggest four ways to reorganize delivery of primary care to meet the challenge of NCDs:

1. Integration of care: shifting from episodic care for discrete symptoms to continuous care for monitoring chronic illness and preventing complications.
2. Innovations in service delivery: task shifting of some primary care services to nonphysicians; active use of treatment guidelines; and adoption of point of care diagnostic technologies.
3. Inclusion of communities and the voice of the patient: including NCD services as essential and reducing financial barriers to access; understanding and incorporating patient preferences in care delivery; and leveraging community and peers to support self-care.
4. Information and communication technologies: exploiting the high penetration of mobile phones in LMICs to promote information sharing and communication of health data in real time.

We have described a variety of promising initiatives in each of these areas under way in middle-income countries. Primary care innovations addressing NCDs are less common in low-income countries, which are constrained by low budgets and still focused on the unfinished infectious disease and maternal/child health agenda. However, in these settings the treatment of HIV—a chronic, communicable disease with many of the same clinical elements and patient experiences as diabetes, heart disease, and asthma—can offer a way to begin reorganizing primary care.[98] Initiatives could be implemented in various settings and adapted to local financial, organizational, and cultural realities.

To make best use of scarce healthcare resources, both financial and human, innovations must improve health and be culturally acceptable and sustainable, which in turn requires robust evaluation. Good evaluation cannot be done without adequate funding and high-level political support. Any evaluation results should be shared with policy and health management communities and not held solely by academics. They should also be shared outside the local health system. Failure to do this leads to best practices being too rarely replicated and failures too often repeated in other countries or even different regions within the same countries. Such sharing of experience has been tried successfully in the area of maternal health and can be adapted to chronic disease.[99]

In theory, primary care is perfectly positioned to take on the challenge of NCDs. As the access point to the health system for people at risk and suffering from NCDs, it is the best platform for screening, diagnosis, and the management and coordination of care. The vast majority of NCD interventions—be they healthy lifestyle counseling, secondary prevention of heart disease through control of hypertension, or palliative oxygen for people with chronic obstructive pulmonary disease—can be delivered by generalist providers. Primary care can also be cost effective: integrating management can save diagnostic and therapeutic costs, and much of the monitoring and routine care can be delegated to nonphysicians.

Despite the abundant evidence of the potential of primary care in addressing NCDs, most developing countries are far from realizing this potential. This shortfall is due to a range of factors, from a concentration of health financing in urban and secondary health facilities to the need to rethink the training of health workers to promote team-based care. On the demand side, populations need more information to modify risky behaviors and to be empowered to demand high-quality care from institutional and individual providers. We have proposed a refocusing of primary care to promote high-quality, integrated, and continuous services that are universally accessible. This reset offers an opportunity to fulfill and expand the vision of Alma Ata in a way that responds to today's health needs and builds a resilient base for tomorrow's health challenges. There is much at stake and much to be gained from implementing and evaluating primary care as a platform for prevention, early detection, diagnosis, disease management, and palliation of chronic and noncommunicable diseases. If primary care can rise to the challenge of chronicity of disease, it will not only save lives and improve health but also potentially strengthen the functioning and responsiveness of entire health systems.

NOTES

The authors are grateful to Dr. Rohini Haar and Ms. Sabrina Hermosilla for their assistance with literature searches and identification of successful examples of primary care NCD approaches.

1. Murray CJL, Vos T, Lozano R, et al. Disability-adjusted life years (DALYs) for 291 diseases and injuries in 21 regions, 1990–2010: a systematic analysis for the Global Burden of Disease Study 2010. *Lancet*. 2012; 380(9859): 2197–2223; Lim SS, Vos T, Flaxman AD, et al. A comparative risk assessment of burden of disease and injury attributable to 67 risk factors and risk factor clusters in 21 regions, 1990–2010: a systematic analysis for the Global Burden of Disease Study 2010. *Lancet*. 2012; 380(9859): 2224–2260.

2. WHO. Global status report on non-communicable diseases 2010. Geneva: World Health Organization; 2011. www.who.int/chp/ncd_global_status_report/en/.

3. Bonita R, Magnusson R, Bovet P, et al. Country actions to meet UN commitments on non-communicable diseases: a stepwise approach. *Lancet*. 2013; 381(9866): 575–584; Murray CJ, Frenk J, Piot P, Mundel T. GBD 2.0: a continuously updated global resource. *Lancet*. 2013; 382(988): 9–11.

4. Murray CJL, Vos T, Lozano R, et al. Disability-adjusted life years (DALYs) for 291 diseases and injuries in 21 regions, 1990–2010: a systematic analysis for the Global Burden of Disease Study 2010. *Lancet*. 2012; 380(9859): 2197–223; WHO. Global status report on noncommunicable diseases 2010. Geneva: World Health Organization; 2011. www.who.int/chp/ncd_global_status_report/en/.

5. WHO. mhGAP: scaling up care for mental, neurological, and substance use disorders. Geneva: World Health Organization; 2008.

6. Beaglehole R, Bonita R, Horton R, et al. Priority actions for the noncommunicable disease crisis. *Lancet*. Apr 23 2011;377(9775):1438–1447.

7. WHO. mhGAP: scaling up care for mental, neurological, and substance use disorders. Geneva: World Health Organization; 2008.

8. Knaul F, Gralow J, Atun R, Bhadelia A. Investing in cancer care and control. In Knaul F, Gralow J R, Atun R, et al., eds. Closing the cancer divide: an equity imperative. Cambridge, MA: Harvard University Press; 2012.

9. Bloom D, Cafiero E, Jane-Llopis E, et al. The global economic burden of noncommunicable diseases. Harvard School of Public Health and World Economic Forum. www.hsph.harvard.edu/pgda/WorkingPapers/2012/PGDA_WP_87.pdf.

10. Beaglehole R, Bonita R, Horton R, et al. Priority actions for the non-communicable disease crisis. *Lancet*. Apr 23 2011;377(9775):1438–1447.

11. United Nations General Assembly. Political Declaration of the High-level Meeting of the General Assembly on the Prevention and Control of Non-communicable Diseases, document A/66/L.1. 2011, www.un.org/ga/search/view_doc.asp?symbol=A /66/L.1.

12. Knaul FM, Bhadelia A, Gralow J, Arreola-Ornelas H, Langer A, Frenk J. Meeting the emerging challenge of breast and cervical cancer in low- and middle-income countries. *Int J Gynaecol Obstet*. 2012;119, Suppl 1:S85–88.

13. Ibrahim MM, Damasceno A. Hypertension in developing countries. *Lancet*. Aug 11 2012;380(9841):611–619.

14. Gakidou E, Mallinger L, Abbott-Klafter J, et al. Management of diabetes and associated cardiovascular risk factors in seven countries: a comparison of data from national health examination surveys. *Bull World Health Organ*. 2011;89(3):172–183.

15. Frenk J, Frejka T, Bobadilla JL, et al. The epidemiologic transition in Latin America. Boletin de la Oficina Sanitaria Panamericana Pan American Sanitary Bureau. 1991;111(6):485–496.

16. McCoy D, Chand S, Sridhar D. Global health funding: how much, where it comes from and where it goes. *Health Policy Plan*. Nov 2009;24(6):407–417.

17. Unal B, Critchley JA, Capewell S. Explaining the decline in coronary heart disease mortality in England and Wales between 1981 and 2000. *Circulation*. Mar 2004;109(9):1101–1107.

18. WHO. Alma-Ata Declaration. Geneva: World Health Organization;1978. Donaldson M, Yordy K, Lohr K, Venselow N, eds. Primary care: America's health in a new era. Washington, DC: National Academies Press; 1996.

19. Beaglehole R, Epping-Jordan J, Patel V, et al. Improving the prevention and management of chronic disease in low-income and middle-income countries: a priority for primary health care. *Lancet*. 2008;372(9642):940–949.

20. De Maeseneer J, Roberts RG, Demarzo M, et al. Tackling NCDs: a different approach is needed. *Lancet*. May 19 2012;379(9829):1860–1861; WHO and World Economic Forum. From burden to "best buys": reducing the economic impact of non-communicable diseases in low- and middle-income countries. Geneva: WHO and World Economic Forum; 2011.

21. WHO. Alma-Ata Declaration. Geneva: WHO; 1978; Atun R, Jaffar S, Nishtar S, et al. Improving responsiveness of health systems to non-communicable diseases. *Lancet*. 2013;381(9867):690–697; Frenk J. Reinventing primary health care: the need for systems integration. *Lancet*. 2009; 374(9684):170–173; Kim JY, Farmer P, Porter ME. Redefining global health-care delivery. *Lancet*. 2013. www.thelancet.com/jour nals/lancet/article/PIIS0140-6736(13)61047-8/fulltext?_eventId=login.

22. Grumbach K. Chronic illness, comorbidities, and the need for medical generalism. *Annals of Family Medicine*. May–Jun 2003;1(1):4–7.

23. Frenk J. Reinventing primary health care: the need for systems integration. *Lancet*. Jul 11 2009;374(9684):170–173.

24. Ibid. See also Smith DL, Bryant JH. Building the infrastructure for primary health care: an overview of vertical and integrated approaches. *Soc Sci Med*. 1988; 26(9):909–917.

25. Nolte E, McKee M. Caring for people with chronic conditions: a health system perspective. Maidenhead, UK: Open University Press; 2008.

26. Ibid.

27. Frenk J. Reinventing primary health care: the need for systems integration. Lancet. 2009;374(9684):170–173.

28. Rabkin M, El-Sadr WM. Why reinvent the wheel? Leveraging the lessons of HIV scale-up to confront non-communicable diseases. *Glob Public Health*. Apr 2011; 6(3):247–256.

29. Ibid.

30. Janssens B, Van Damme W, Raleigh B, et al. Offering integrated care for HIV/AIDS, diabetes and hypertension within chronic disease clinics in Cambodia. *Bull World Health Organ*. Nov 2007;85(11):880–885.

31. Macinko J, Marinho de Souza Mde F, Guanais FC, da Silva Simoes CC. Going to scale with community-based primary care: an analysis of the family health program and infant mortality in Brazil, 1999–2004. *Soc Sci Med*. 2007;65(10):2070–80; Unger J-P, De Paepe P, Buitron R, Soors W. Costa Rica: achievements of a heterodox health policy. Am J Public Health. 2008; 98(4): 636–643; Knaul FM, Gonzalez-Pier E, Gomez-Dantes O, et al. The quest for universal health coverage: achieving social protection for all in Mexico. *Lancet*. 2012;380(9849):1259–79.

32. Mendonca CS, Harzheim E, Duncan BB, Nunes LN, Leyh W. Trends in hospitalizations for primary care sensitive conditions following the implementation of Family Health Teams in Belo Horizonte, Brazil. *Health Policy and Planning*. July 2012;27(4):348–355. See also Ministério da Saúde. *Política Nacional de Promocao da Saúde*. Brasilia; 2010.

33. Instituto Nacional De Cancerologia. 2012; www.incan.edu.mx/.

34. Chen L, Evans T, Anand S, et al. Human resources for health: overcoming the crisis. *Lancet*. Nov 27–Dec 3 2004;364(9449):1984–1990; Frenk J, Chen L, Bhutta ZA, et al. Health professionals for a new century: transforming education to strengthen health systems in an interdependent world. *Lancet*. 2010;376(9756):1923–1958.

35. WHO. World Health Report 2006: working together for health. Geneva: World Health Organization; 2006.

36. Lekoubou A, Awah P, Fezeu L, Sobngwi E, Kengne AP. Hypertension, diabetes mellitus and task shifting their management in sub-Saharan Africa. *Int J Environ Res Public Health*. Feb 2010;7(2):353–363; Lehmann U, Van Damme W, Barten F, Sanders D. Task shifting: the answer to the human resources crisis in Africa? *Hum Resour Health*. 2009;7:49.

37. Kruk ME, Pereira C, Vaz F, Bergstrom S, Galea S. Economic evaluation of surgically trained assistant medical officers in performing major obstetric surgery in Mozambique. *BJOG*. Oct 2007;114(10):1253–1260; Pereira C, Cumbi A, Malalane R, et al. Meeting the need for emergency obstetric care in Mozambique: work performance

and histories of medical doctors and assistant medical officers trained for surgery. *BJOG*. Dec 2007;114(12):1530–1533; Chilopora G, Pereira C, Kamwendo F, Chimbiri A, Malunga E, Bergstrom S. Postoperative outcome of caesarean sections and other major emergency obstetric surgery by clinical officers and medical officers in Malawi. *Human Resources for Health*. 2007;5(1):17; McCord C, Mbaruku G, Pereira C, Nzabu- hakwa C, Bergstrom S. The quality of emergency obstetrical surgery by assistant medical officers in Tanzanian district hospitals. *Health Aff* (Millwood). Sep–Oct 2009;28(5):w876–885.

38. Pereira C, Cumbi A, Malalane R, et al. Meeting the need for emergency ob- stetric care in Mozambique: work performance and histories of medical doctors and assistant medical officers trained for surgery. *BJOG*. Dec 2007;114(12):1530–1533.

39. McCord C, Mbaruku G, Pereira C, Nzabuhakwa C, Bergstrom S. The quality of emergency obstetrical surgery by assistant medical officers in Tanzanian district hospitals. *Health Aff* (Millwood). Sep–Oct 2009;28(5):w876–885; Yu D, Souteyrand Y, Banda MA, Kaufman J, Perriens JH. Investment in HIV/AIDS programs: does it help strengthen health systems in developing countries? *Globalization and Health*. 2008;4(8):8; Fairall L, Bachmann MO, Lombard C, et al. Task shifting of antiretro- viral treatment from doctors to primary-care nurses in South Africa (STRETCH): a pragmatic, parallel, cluster-randomised trial. *Lancet*. Sep 2012;380(9845):889–898; Mdege ND, Chindove S, et al. The effectiveness and cost implications of task-shifting in the delivery of antiretroviral therapy to HIV-infected patients: a systematic review. *Health policy and planning*. 2013;28(3):223–236.

40. Adams JL, Almond ML, Ringo EJ, Shangali WH, Sikkema KJ. Feasibility of nurse-led antidepressant medication management of depression in an HIV clinic in Tanzania. *Int J Psychiatry Med*. 2012;43(2):105–117; Labhardt ND, Balo JR, et al. Im- proved retention rates with low-cost interventions in hypertension and diabetes management in a rural African environment of nurse-led care: a cluster-randomised trial. *Tropical medicine & international health*. 2011;16(10):1276–1284.

41. Kengne AP, Awah PK, Fezeu LL, Sobngwi E, Mbanya JC. Primary health care for hypertension by nurses in rural and urban sub-Saharan Africa. *J Clin Hypertens* (Green- wich). Oct 2009;11(10):564–572; Kengne AP, Fezeu L, Sobngwi E, et al. Type 2 diabetes management in nurse-led primary healthcare settings in urban and rural Cameroon. *Prim Care Diabetes*. Aug 2009;3(3):181–188; Kengne AP, Sobngwi E, Fezeu LL, Awah PK, Dongmo S, Mbanya JC. Nurse-led care for asthma at primary level in rural sub-Saharan Africa: the experience of Bafut in Cameroon. *J Asthma*. Aug 2008;45(6):437–443.

42. De Maeseneer J, Roberts RG, Demarzo M, et al. Tackling NCDs: a different approach is needed. *Lancet*. May 19 2012;379(9829):1860–1861.

43. Ibid.; see also Mdege ND, Chindove S, Ali S. The effectiveness and cost im- plications of task-shifting in the delivery of antiretroviral therapy to HIV-infected patients: a systematic review. *Health Policy Plan*. Jun 2012:223–236.

44. Abegunde DO, Shengelia B, Luyten A, et al. Can non-physician health-care workers assess and manage cardiovascular risk in primary care? *Bull World Health Organ*. 2007;85(6):432–440.

45. Kar SS, Thakur J, Jain S, Kumar R. Cardiovascular disease risk management in a primary health care setting of north India. *Indian Heart Journal*. 2008;60(1):19.

46. Wagner EH, Austin BT, Von Korff M. Organizing care for patients with chronic illness. *Milbank Quarterly*. 1996;74(4):511–544.

47. Barcelo A, Cafiero E, de Boer M, et al. Using collaborative learning to improve diabetes care and outcomes: the VIDA project. *Prim Care Diabetes*. Oct 2010; 4(3):145–153.

48. Ministerio de Salud. 2012; www.remediar.gov.ar/.

49. Chamie G, Kwarisiima D, Clark TD, et al. Leveraging rapid community-based HIV testing campaigns for non-communicable diseases in rural Uganda. *PLoS One*. 2012;7(8):e43400.

50. Ibid.

51. Denny L, Kuhn L, De Souza M, Pollack AE, Dupree W, Wright TC, Jr. Screen-and-treat approaches for cervical cancer prevention in low-resource settings: a randomized controlled trial. *JAMA*. Nov 2005;294(17):2173–2181; Luciani S, Munoz S, Gonzales M, Delgado JM, Valcarcel M. Effectiveness of cervical cancer screening using visual inspection with acetic acid in Peru. *Int J Gynaecol Obstet*. Oct 2011;115(1):53–56.

52. Ibrahim A, Aro AR, Rasch V, Pukkala E. Cervical cancer screening in primary health care setting in Sudan: a comparative study of visual inspection with acetic acid and Pap smear. *Int J Women's Health*. 2012;4:67–73; Audet CM, Silva Matos C, Blevins M, Cardoso A, Moon TD, Sidat M. Acceptability of cervical cancer screening in rural Mozambique. *Health Educ Res*. Jun 2012;27(3):544–551; Li R, Lewkowitz AK, Zhao FH, et al. Analysis of the effectiveness of visual inspection with acetic acid / Lugol's iodine in one-time and annual follow-up screening in rural China. *Arch Gynecol Obstet*. Jun 2012;285(6):1627–1632; Ramogola-Masire D, de Klerk R, Monare B, Ratshaa B, Friedman HM, Zetola NM. Cervical cancer prevention in HIV-infected women using the "see and treat" approach in Botswana. *J Acquir Immune Defic Syndr*. Mar 2012;59(3):308–313.

53. Salvador-Davila G, Gaffikin L. Bringing cervical cancer detection and early treatment closer to women: a Peruvian experience (1996–2000). Baltimore: JH-PIEGO, June 2003; http://screening.iarc.fr/doc/cecap03peresults.pdf; Schweninger E. The Peruvian League in the fight against cancer: mobile detection units. Center for Health Market Innovations, 2011; http://healthmarketinnovations.org/sites/healthmarketinnovations.org/files/LPLCC_CaseStudy_0.pdf.

54. Gupta R. Smoking, educational status and health inequity in India. *Indian J. Med. Res.* Jul 2006;124(1):15–22; Mayosi BM, Flisher AJ, Lalloo UG, Sitas F, Tollman SM, Bradshaw D. The burden of non-communicable diseases in South Africa. *Lancet*. Sep 12 2009;374(9693):934–947; DeSantis C, Siegel R, Bandi P, Jemal A. Breast cancer statistics, 2011. *CA Cancer J Clin*. Nov–Dec 2011;61(6):409–418; Bleich SN, Jarlenski MP, Bell CN, LaVeist TA. Health inequalities: trends, progress, and policy. *Annu Rev Public Health*. Apr 2012;33:7–40.

55. Kruk ME, Goldmann E, Galea S. Borrowing and selling to pay for health care in low- and middle-income countries. *Health Aff* (Millwood). Jul–Aug 2009;

28(4):1056–1066; McIntyre D, Thiede M, Birch S. Access as a policy-relevant concept in low- and middle-income countries. *Health Econ Policy Law.* Jan 30 2009;4:179–193; Knaul FM, Wong R, Arreola-Ornelas H, Pleic M. Introduction. In Knaul FM, Wong R, Arreola-Ornelas H, eds. Household spending and impoverishment. Cambridge, MA: Global Equity Initiative and Harvard University Press, 2013.

56. Nabyonga J, Desmet M, Karamagi H, Kadama P, Omaswa F, Walker O. Abolition of cost-sharing is pro-poor: evidence from Uganda. *Health Policy Plan.* March 2005;20(2):100–108; Lagarde M, Palmer N. The impact of user fees on access to health services in low- and middle-income countries. *Cochrane Database Syst Rev.* 2011(4):CD009094; Lagarde M, Barroy H, Palmer N. Assessing the effects of removing user fees in Zambia and Niger. *J Health Serv Res Policy.* Jan 2012;17(1):30–36.

57. Hall V, Thomsen RW, Henriksen O, Lohse N. Diabetes in sub-Saharan Africa 1999–2011: epidemiology and public health implications. A systematic review. *BMC Public Health.* 2011;11:564.

58. Labhardt ND, Balo JR, Ndam M, Manga E, Stoll B. Improved retention rates with low-cost interventions in hypertension and diabetes management in a rural African environment of nurse-led care: a cluster-randomised trial. *Trop Med Int Health.* Jul 2011:1276–1284.

59. Frenk J. Reinventing primary health care: the need for systems integration. *Lancet.* Jul 11 2009;374(9684):170–173.

60. Cerdas M. Epidemiology and control of hypertension and diabetes in Costa Rica. *Ren Fail.* 2006;28(8):693–696.

61. Arredondo A, Zuniga A. Epidemiological changes and financial consequences of hypertension in Latin America: implications for the health system and patients in Mexico. *Cad. Saude Publica.* Mar 2012;28(3):497–502.

62. Fernald LC, Hou X, Gertler PJ. Oportunidades program participation and body mass index, blood pressure, and self-reported health in Mexican adults. *Prev Chronic Dis.* Jul 2008;5(3):A81.

63. Holman H, Lorig K. Patients as partners in managing chronic disease: partnership is a prerequisite for effective and efficient health care. *BMJ.* Feb 26 2000;320(7234):526–527.

64. WHO. Noncommunicable Diseases and Mental Health Cluster. Innovative care for chronic conditions: building blocks for actions: global report. Geneva: World Health Organization; 2002.

65. Frenk J. Reinventing primary health care: the need for systems integration. *Lancet.* Jul 11 2009;374(9684):170–173.

66. WHO. World Health Report 2000. Health systems: improving performance. Geneva: WHO, 2000. www.who.int/whr/2000/en/whr00_en.pdf.

67. Cheraghi-Sohi S, Hole AR, Mead N, et al. What patients want from primary care consultations: a discrete choice experiment to identify patients' priorities. *Ann Fam Med.* Mar–Apr 2008;6(2):107–115; Gyrd-Hansen D, Sogaard J. Analysing public preferences for cancer screening programmes. *Health Econ.* Oct 2001;10(7):617–634;

Kruk ME, Paczkowski M, Mbaruku G, de Pinho H, Galea S. Women's preferences for place of delivery in rural Tanzania: a population-based discrete choice experiment. *Am J Public Health*. Sep 2009;99(9):1666–1672; Kruk, ME, Rockers PC, et al. Population preferences for health care in Liberia: insights for rebuilding a health system. *Health services research* 2011;46(6pt2):2057–2078; Rubin G, Bate A, George A, Shackley P, Hall N. Preferences for access to the GP: a discrete choice experiment. *Br J Gen Pract*. Oct 2006;56(531):743–748.

68. Cheraghi-Sohi S, Hole AR, Mead N, et al. What patients want from primary care consultations: a discrete choice experiment to identify patients' priorities. *Ann Fam Med*. Mar–Apr 2008;6(2):107–115.

69. Nolte E, McKee M. Caring for people with chronic conditions: a health system perspective. Maidenhead, UK: Open University Press; 2008.

70. WHO. Noncommunicable Diseases and Mental Health Cluster. Innovative care for chronic conditions: building blocks for actions: global report. Geneva: World Health Organization; 2002.

71. Funnell MM. Peer-based behavioural strategies to improve chronic disease self-management and clinical outcomes: evidence, logistics, evaluation considerations and needs for future research. *Fam Pract*. Jun 2010;27, Suppl 1:i17–22; Heisler M. Different models to mobilize peer support to improve diabetes self-management and clinical outcomes: evidence, logistics, evaluation considerations and needs for future research. *Fam Pract*. Jun 2010;27, Suppl 1:i23–32.

72. Brownstein JN, Chowdhury FM, Norris SL, et al. Effectiveness of community health workers in the care of people with hypertension. *Am J Prev Med*. May 2007;32(5):435–447.

73. Norris SL, Chowdhury FM, Van Le K, et al. Effectiveness of community health workers in the care of persons with diabetes. *Diabet Med*. May 2006;23(5):544–556.

74. Prince M, Acosta D, Albanese E, et al. Ageing and dementia in low and middle income countries—using research to engage with public and policy makers. *International Review of Psychiatry*. 2008;20(4):332–343.

75. Celletti F, Wright A, Palen J, et al. Can the deployment of community health workers for the delivery of HIV services represent an effective and sustainable response to health workforce shortages? Results of a multicountry study. *Aids*. Jan 2010;24, Suppl 1:S45–57.

76. Fu D, Fu H, McGowan P, et al. Implementation and quantitative evaluation of chronic disease self-management programme in Shanghai, China: randomized controlled trial. *Bull World Health Organ*. 2003;81(3):174–182.

77. Wringe A, Cataldo F, Stevenson N, Fakoya A. Delivering comprehensive home-based care programmes for HIV: a review of lessons learned and challenges ahead in the era of antiretroviral therapy. *Health Policy Plan*. Sep 2010;25(5):352–362.

78. Lorig K, Holman H. Arthritis self-management studies: a twelve-year review. *Health Education Quarterly*. 1993;20:17–28.

79. Coomes CM, Lewis MA, Uhrig JD, Furberg RD, Harris JL, Bann CM. Beyond reminders: a conceptual framework for using short message service to promote

prevention and improve healthcare quality and clinical outcomes for people living with HIV. *AIDS Care.* 2012;24(3):348–357.

80. Kahn JG, Yang JS, Kahn JS. "Mobile" health needs and opportunities in developing countries. *Health Aff* (Millwood). Feb 2010;29(2):252–258. By 2013, the International Telecommunications Union estimated 6.8 billion mobile phone subscriptions—nearly one for every person on the planet; The world in 2013: ICT facts and figures. Geneva: International Telecommunication Union; February 2013; www.itu.int/en/ITU-D/Statistics/Documents/facts/ICTFactsFigures2013.pdf.

81. Piette JD, Lun KC, Moura LA, Jr., et al. Impacts of e-health on the outcomes of care in low- and middle-income countries: where do we go from here? *Bull World Health Organ.* May 2012;90(5):365–372.

82. Miron-Shatz T, Ratzan SC. The potential of an online and mobile health scorecard for preventing chronic disease. *J Health Commun.* Aug 2011;16 Suppl 2:175–190; Ekeland AG, Bowes A, Flottorp S. Effectiveness of telemedicine: a systematic review of reviews. *Int J Med Inform.* Nov 2010;79(11):736–771; Blaya JA, Fraser HS, Holt B. E-health technologies show promise in developing countries. *Health Aff* (Millwood). Feb 2010;29(2):244–251.

83. Cole-Lewis H, Kershaw T. Text messaging as a tool for behavior change in disease prevention and management. *Epidemiol Rev.* Apr 2010;32(1):56–69.

84. Fjeldsoe BS, Marshall AL, Miller YD. Behavior change interventions delivered by mobile telephone short-message service. *Am J Prev Med.* Feb 2009;36(2):165–173; Wei J, Hollin I, Kachnowski S. A review of the use of mobile phone text messaging in clinical and healthy behaviour interventions. *J Telemed Telecare.* 2011;17(1):41–48.

85. Car J, Gurol-Urganci I, de Jongh T, Vodopivec-Jamsek V, Atun R. Mobile phone messaging reminders for attendance at healthcare appointments. *Cochrane Database Syst Rev.* 2012;7:CD007458; Guy R, Hocking J, Wand H, Stott S, Ali H, Kaldor J. How effective are short message service reminders at increasing clinic attendance? A meta-analysis and systematic review. *Health Serv Res.* Apr 2012;47(2):614–632.

86. Liang X, Wang Q, Yang X, et al. Effect of mobile phone intervention for diabetes on glycaemic control: a meta-analysis. *Diabet Med.* Apr 2011;28(4):455–463.

87. Whittaker R, Borland R, Bullen C, Lin RB, McRobbie H, Rodgers A. Mobile phone-based interventions for smoking cessation. *Cochrane Database Syst Rev.* 2009(4):CD006611.

88. Free C, Knight R, Robertson S, et al. Smoking cessation support delivered via mobile phone text messaging (txt2stop): a single-blind, randomised trial. *Lancet.* Jul 2 2011;378(9785):49–55.

89. Horvath T, Azman H, Kennedy GE, Rutherford GW. Mobile phone text messaging for promoting adherence to antiretroviral therapy in patients with HIV infection. *Cochrane Database Syst Rev.* 2012;3:CD009756.

90. Piette JD, Mendoza-Avelares MO, Milton EC, Lange I, Fajardo R. Access to mobile communication technology and willingness to participate in automated telemedicine calls among chronically ill patients in Honduras. *Telemedicine Journal and*

e-health. Dec 2010;16(10):1030–1041; Piette JD, Mendoza-Avelares MO, Ganser M, Mohamed M, Marinec N, Krishnan S. A preliminary study of a cloud-computing model for chronic illness self-care support in an underdeveloped country. *Am J Prev Med.* Jun 2011;40(6):629–632.

91. Kahn JG, Yang JS, Kahn JS. "Mobile" health needs and opportunities in developing countries. *Health Aff* (Millwood). Feb 2010;29(2):252–258; van Olmen J, Ku GM, Bermejo R, Kegels G, Hermann K, Van Damme W. The growing caseload of chronic life-long conditions calls for a move towards full self-management in low-income countries. *Globalization and Health.* 2011;7(1):38; Deglise C, Suggs LS, Odermatt P. Short message service (SMS) applications for disease prevention in developing countries. *J Med Internet Res.* 2012;14(1):e3.

92. Frenk J, Gonzalez-Pier E, Gomez-Dantes O, Lezana MA, Knaul FM. Comprehensive reform to improve health system performance in Mexico. *Lancet.* 2006; 368:1524–1534; King G, Gakidou E, Imai K, et al. Public policy for the poor? A randomised assessment of the Mexican universal health insurance programme. *Lancet.* Apr 25 2009;373(9673):1447–1454; Knaul FM, Arreola-Ornelas H, Mendez-Carniado O, et al. Evidence is good for your health system: policy reform to remedy catastrophic and impoverishing health spending in Mexico. *Lancet.* Nov 18 2006;368(9549):1828–1841; Victora CG, Peters DH. Seguro popular in Mexico: is premature evaluation healthy? *Lancet.* Apr 25 2009;373(9673):1404–1405.

93. Victora CG, Schellenberg JA, Huicho L, et al. Context matters: interpreting impact findings in child survival evaluations. *Health Policy Plan.* Dec 2005;20(1), Suppl 1:i18–i31.

94. Walker A, Grimshaw J, Johnston M, Pitts N, Steen N, Eccles M. PRIME— PRocess modelling in ImpleMEntation research: selecting a theoretical basis for interventions to change clinical practice. *BMC Health Services Research.* 2003;3(1):22; Madon T, Hofman KJ, Kupfer L, Glass RI. Public health: implementation science. *Science.* December 2007;318(5857):1728–1729.

95. Greenhalgh T, Robert G, Macfarlane F, Bate P, Kyriakidou O. Diffusion of innovations in service organizations: systematic review and recommendations. *Milbank Quarterly.* 2004;82:581–629; Damschroder L, Aron D, Keith R, Kirsh S, Alexander J, Lowery J. Fostering implementation of health services research findings into practice: a consolidated framework for advancing implementation science. *Implementation Science.* 2009;4(1):50; Azad K, Barnett S, Banerjee B, et al. Effect of scaling up women's groups on birth outcomes in three rural districts in Bangladesh: a cluster-randomised controlled trial. *Lancet.* Apr 3 2010;375(9721):1193–1202.

96. WHO. *Global status report on non-communicable diseases 2010.* Geneva: World Health Organization; 2011.

97. Beaglehole R, Epping-Jordan J, Patel V, et al. Improving the prevention and management of chronic disease in low-income and middle-income countries: a priority for primary health care. *Lancet.* 2008;372(9642):940–949; Frenk J. Reinventing primary health care: the need for systems integration. *Lancet.* Jul 11 2009;374(9684):170–173.

98. Rabkin M, El-Sadr WM. Why reinvent the wheel? Leveraging the lessons of HIV scale-up to confront non-communicable diseases. *Global Public Health*. Apr 2011;6(3):247–256.

99. WHO. Morocco Maternal Mortality Forum. Geneva: World Health Organization; 2011, www.who.int/pmnch/media/membernews/2011/20110629_morocco _forum/en/index.html.

CHAPTER 5

Sectoral Cooperation for the Prevention and Control of NCDs

George Alleyne and Sania Nishtar

This chapter will explicate the nature of and possibilities for the sectoral cooperation that is necessary for health and of particular relevance to non-communicable diseases. It will examine the notion and possibilities of this co-operation beginning with the Political Declaration (PD) from the September 2011 United Nations High-level Meeting (HLM) on the Prevention and Control of Non-communicable Diseases.[1] It will give some of the historical and theoretical background as a basis for explaining the approaches that need to be considered in the operationalization of the mandates of the PD. Its central thesis is that there is a fundamental difference between multisectoral and intersectoral coop-eration. The former embraces cooperation among agencies of the government while the latter expresses the relationship among the three key sectors of the state—the government, the private sector, and civil society. This difference is important in structuring an appropriate response to NCDs, as is called for in the PD.

The Context: The Political Declaration on NCDs

The major social problems of our time are by definition complex and certainly, in democratic societies, the only hope of addressing them is by the involvement of many parts of society. Difficult though collaboration may be, there is no other option. Health is one such complex social field, and the threat that NCDs pose to that health has been well described in the literature.

The more compelling reasons relate to mortality and morbidity and the economic as well as the social effects of NCDs. They are now the leading causes of death globally. The World Health Organization estimates that 80% of deaths in the low- and middle-income countries are due to NCDs. In 2008, almost two-thirds of the 57 million deaths were due to NCDs, and it is a tragic datum that one-quarter of NCD-related deaths occur in adults below the age of sixty years.[2] It is estimated that in the next two decades, NCDs will cost more than US$ 30 trillion.[3] NCDs not only cause poverty but occur more frequently in the poor and prevent them from escaping from the poverty trap. The gender dimension is also being recognized, as much of the chronic care of persons with NCDs falls on women and girls, thus preventing them from acquiring the education necessary for them to be optimally productive citizens.

It is not surprising, therefore, that discussions at high political levels addressing NCDs would emphasize the critical need for multisectoriality. The term "multisectoral" was mentioned 15 times in the PD. Not only was it mentioned frequently, but it occurs in several different contexts. The opening paragraph under the heading of "Responding to the challenge: a whole-of-government and a whole-of-society approach" establishes the framework for a multisectoral approach. Paragraph 33 states: "Recognize that the rising prevalence, morbidity and mortality of non-communicable disease worldwide, can be largely prevented and controlled through collective and multisectoral action by all Member States and other relevant stakeholders at local, national, regional and global levels, and by raising the priority accorded to noncomunicable disease in development cooperation by enhancing such cooperation in this regard."

Thus there is a call for sectoral cooperation at the government level, and the possible actors at that level are spelled out in paragraph 36 of the PD by naming the possible sectors—health, education, energy, agriculture, sports, transport, communication, urban planning, environment, labor, employment, industry and trade, finance, and social and economic development. In addition, the stakeholders that might represent sectors at the level of society are also spelled out and are said to include "individuals, families and communities, intergovernmental organizations and religious institutions, civil society, academia, media, voluntary associations." It is important to note that the private sector and industry are mentioned in this context.

In further mentions of the multisectoral approach, the PD refers to the many arrangements to be made under this rubric—engagement, efforts, actions, approaches, and interventions. In relation to national and public policies, it emphasized that the effective response had to be multisectoral as well. The PD also calls for the Secretary General to present "options for strengthening and facilitating multisectoral action for the prevention and control of NCDs through effective partnership" (paragraph 64). The World Health Organization has been engaged in an active process of consultation on the form and functioning of such multisectoral action,[4] and the Executive Board in its 2012 session resolved that explicit options for facilitating multisectoral action through effective partnerships be outlined as a priority.[5]

The PD emphasized the importance of multisectoral action for *governments* in a number of ways, foremost by espousing the "whole of government" principle and the notion of "health in all policies" directly, but also by calling for multisectoral national policies and national plans for NCDs, the integration of NCDs in national development agendas. The declaration also consistently referred to a level of leadership in its language, which pitched responsibility at a much higher level than ministries of health.

Through its endorsement of the 2000 Global Strategy for the Prevention and Control of NCDs and reiteration of the need to accelerate implementation of certain WHO normative frameworks, it grounded its *international development approach* to NCDs in multisectoral action. These frameworks, namely, the WHO Framework Convention on Tobacco Control, the Global Strategy on Diet, Physical Activity and Health, and the Global Strategy to Reduce the Harmful Effects of Alcohol, cannot be implemented without action outside of the health sector. Most of the strategies called for have been included in a core set of multisectoral interventions, the evidence-based "best buys," which the WHO regards as a priority to be brought to scale. The PD cast NCDs as wide as possible in the international development context by recalling the threat NCDs pose for social and economic development and reiterating the need for their inclusion in global development agendas. Additionally, its support for instruments such as multidonor trust funds and platforms for North-South and South-South cooperation call for broad-based development engagement, both domestically as well as globally.

In outlining the linkages of NCDs with maternal and child health, in terms of risks, and HIV/AIDS, in terms of health systems integration, in order to form an effective response, another dimension of multisectoral action has been referred to as one in which vertical public health streams can be considered as "sectors." This is relevant both for domestic and international planning.

The PD's emphasis on multisectoral action was also evident in its support for multisectoral frameworks for planning, monitoring, and evaluation and its articulation of targets, which necessitate action outside the arena of health. Through an explicit reference to the universal coverage goals, it linked the NCD agenda with the labor and insurance "markets," social protection systems, human rights and health security, aid effectiveness, bottom-of-pyramid initiatives, and public-private partnership agendas. Each of these areas belongs to a different sector.

The PD was not the first international normative instrument to emphasize the notion of multisectoriality. This was in evidence in many of the fora leading up to the UN HLM. The Caribbean heads of government, in their historic 2007 summit in Port-of-Spain on prevention and control of NCDs, issued a 15-point declaration that emphasized multisectoral action: "the burdens of NCDs can be reduced by comprehensive and integrated preventive and control strategies at the individual, family, community, national and regional levels and through collaborative programmes, partnerships and policies supported by governments, private sectors, NGOs and our other social, regional and international partners." It also called for establishing multisectoral national commissions.[6]

Similarly, in 2009, the 54 Commonwealth Heads of Government in calling for a UN Summit on NCDs stressed the importance of sectoral cooperation as follows: "We firmly believe that the incidence and burdens of NCDs can be reduced through comprehensive and integrated preventive and control strategies at the individual, family, community, national and regional levels and through collaborative programmes, partnerships and policies supported by governments, the private sector, NGOs and our other social, regional and international partners. We therefore call for global engagement of the private sector, civil society and governments in efforts to combat these diseases."

International instruments other than the PD that referred to and emphasized the notion of multisectoral action are summarized in box 5.1.

Box 5.1 International Instruments and Multisectoral Action

Declaration of the Heads of State and Government of the Caribbean Community, "Uniting to stop the epidemic of chronic non-communicable diseases"[a]
Libreville Declaration on Health and Environment in Africa[b]
The statement of the Commonwealth Heads of Government on action to combat noncommunicable diseases[c]
The outcome declaration of the Fifth Summit of the Americas
Parma Declaration on Environment and Health, adopted by the member states in the WHO European Region
Dubai Declaration on Diabetes and Chronic Non-communicable Diseases in the Middle East and Northern Africa Region
European Charter on Counteracting Obesity
Aruban Call for Action on Obesity
Honiara Communiqué on addressing noncommunicable disease challenges in the Pacific region
Ministerial Declaration adopted at the 2009 high-level segment of the UN Economic and Social Council Resolution 65/238
WHO Framework Convention on Tobacco Control[d]
WHO Global Strategy on Diet and Physical Activity
World Health Assembly document: Prevention and control of noncommunicable diseases: implementation of the global strategy[e]
Negotiated agreements for the reduction of salt in processed food[f,g]
Policy statements of bilateral development agencies[h,i]
Institute of Medicine report: Recommendations of the Committee on the U.S. Commitment to Global Health[j]
World Bank report: Public policy and the challenge of chronic non-communicable diseases[k]
Ouagadougou Declaration on Primary Health Care and health systems in Africa[l]
The Kampala Declaration and Agenda for Global Action[m]
Address of permanent Mission of Qatar to the UN, President of the Economic and Social Council[n]

---

[a] Caribbean Community (CARICOM) Secretariat. Georgetown, Guyana: CARICOM. www.caricom.org/jsp /communications/meetings_statements/declaration_port_of_spain_chronic_ncds.jsp. Accessed May 11, 2012.

[b] Health Security through healthy environments. First inter-ministerial conference on health in Asia. www.unep.org/health-env/pdfs/libreville-declaration-eng.pdf. Accessed May 11, 2012.

[c] Commonwealth Secretariat. Proceedings of the Commonwealth Heads of Government meeting: 2009 November 27–29; Port-of-Spain, Trinidad and Tobago. London, 2010. www.thecommonwealth.org/files /232640/FileName/CHOGM_Outcome-Docs_Communique_09_PRINT.pdf.

[d] World Health Organization. Conference of the parties to the WHO framework convention on tobacco control (document repository): www.who.int/gb/fctc/. Accessed May 20, 2012.

[e] World Health Organization. World Health Assembly document A61/8. www.who.int/gb/ebwha/pdf _files/A61/A61_8-en.pdf. Accessed May 20, 2010.

(continued)

Box 5.1 (*continued*)

  f World Health Organization.World Action on Salt and Health. www.worldactiononsalt.com/. Accessed May 20, 2012.
  g World Health Organization. Reducing salt intake in populations: report of a WHO forum and technical meeting. Geneva: WHO; 2007.
  h UK Department for International Development. Working together for better health DFID health strategy, 2007. www.dfid.gov.uk/pubs/files/health-strategy07.pdf.
  i Australian Agency for International Development. Helping health systems deliver. A policy for Australian Development Assistance in Health. Canberra: AusAID; 2006.
  j Institute of Medicine. The US Commitment to Global Health: recommendations for the Public and Private Sectors. Washington, DC: National Academies Press; 2009.
  k Adeyi O, Smith O, Robles S. Washington, DC: World Bank; 2005.
  l World Health Organization. Ouagadougou Declaration on primary health care and health systems in Africa: achieving better health for Africa in the new millennium: Burkina Faso, 28–30 April 2008. www.afro .who.int/phc_hs_2008/documents/En/Ouagadougou%20declaration%20version%20Eng.pdf.
  m World Health Organization. Global Workforce Alliance. www.ghwa.org/. Accessed May 20, 2012. www .who.int/gb/ebwha/pdf_files/A61/A61_8-en.pdf. Accessed May 20, 2012.
  n Note Verbale dated June 2009. www.un.org/ecosoc/newfunct/pdf/Qatar%20-%20Report%20of %20the%20Western%20Asia%20regional%20preparatory%20meeting%20-%20Version%2025%20June %202009%20at%2010AM.pdf.

Multisectoral and Intersectoral Approaches

The term *sector* is used in many different ways. As a notion, *sector* gained prominence in parallel with the evolution of approaches to aid disbursement by international financial institutions. Sector Wide Approaches were fraught with challenges and led to intrasectoral and intersectoral imbalances, which resulted in the birth of the Programme Assistance Approach and later the on-budget approach to aid. However, more recently the World Bank has introduced a new instrument— Program-for-Results—to advance development effectiveness.[7] According to the Bank, "The instrument will focus on development results by linking disbursements to results or performance indicators, which can be outputs, outcomes, or other actions/results that are tangible, transparent, and verifiable. Program-for-Results will work directly with the program's institutions and systems and will seek to strengthen those institutions' governance, capacities, and systems over time." While not specifically designed for this purpose, it is possible that the instrument will facilitate both multisectoral and intersectoral cooperation.

In this chapter, the term *sector* is understood in the social sense as a distinct subset of a market, society, industry, or economy where components share similar characteristics. We assume that the term *multisectoral* was used in the PD deliberately, but some contexts in which it was used indicate that the concept of intersectoriality was more appropriate. The terms *multisectoral* and *intersectoral* are

often used interchangeably. This is unfortunate, as in our view there are fundamental differences in the two approaches and indeed, some of the approaches
recommended in the PD do not fall into the single category of multisectorality
but fall into either category. Thus it is useful to examine more closely the origins
and development of sectoral cooperation in health. The possible differences are
not merely epistemological niceties but represent fundamentally different approaches to structuring the potential solutions to health problems in general and
NCDs in particular.

Both approaches can be described as essentially a form of partnership. Bryson
et al. give a useful characterization of such partnerships. They describe a continuum, at one end of which we find organizations or sectors existing almost in
isolation, with hardly any contact between or among them. At the other end,
they fuse so intimately as to result in the formation of almost a completely new
entity that takes on a character in which authorities and capabilities are merged.[8]
Most arrangements are somewhere along this continuum. A multisectoral arrangement would tend toward the isolation end of the continuum, while an intersectoral
one would find itself toward the merged end of the continuum.

Multisectoral Cooperation
Defining Multisectoral Cooperation

It is possible to define multisectoral cooperation as cooperation in which sectors
maintain their identity and each approaches the problem from the perspective of
their own agency and with the use of their own resources. This is the more common situation within government, in which sectors are usually within the
administrative and political responsibility of a ministry or other government institution. In practice, sector "B" assists sector "A" with the solution to a problem
that, strictly speaking, is not within the mandate of sector B. Because political
kudos often go to the accomplishments of one particular sector, there is no intrinsic drive for sector B to assist sector A. And given that resources are allocated
strictly according to sectors in most governments, there is even less motive for
one sector to devote its resources to solving or addressing a problem that is the
responsibility of another sector. Because of the public perception that the health
sector is responsible for "delivering health," there is a parochial interest on the
part of the health sector in solving those problems that impact health but whose
solutions lie outside the purview of the health sector.

One may describe two forms of interest. There is intrinsic parochial interest
peculiar to the sector, and there are liberal interests shared by all who have some

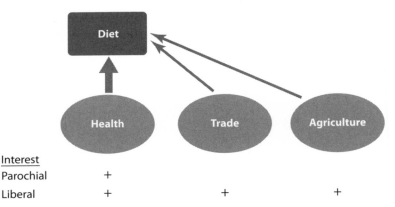

Interest			
Parochial	+		
Liberal	+	+	+

Fig. 5.1. The multisectoral approach, with diet as an example. The health sector has a parochial as well as a liberal interest in diet as one of the risk factors for NCDs. The other sectors have only a general or liberal interest in the health aspect of diet.

stake in the public welfare. It is fair to assume that all members of a government share a common interest in its particular approach to enhancing public welfare. Thus the health sector has both parochial as well as liberal interest, while the transport sector, for example, whose actions bear on the health of the public, has a liberal interest in health but has no parochial interest or responsibility (fig. 5.1). The education sector may be an exception, in that health may represent both a parochial as well as a liberal interest (see Box 5.2).

Stimulating Multisectoral Cooperation

Multisectoral cooperation usually arises when the solution of the particular problem is a matter of national interest to such an extent that it becomes national rather than sectoral policy, and the interests of all possible contributing sectors are stimulated from a level above that of the sectoral heads. The head of state or prime minister, through the cabinet process or directly, indicates that there must be cooperation among or between sectors. Multisectoral cooperation can also be stimulated by pressure from civil society emphasizing the relevance of the extra-sectoral issue to the sector in question.

Some maintain that multisectoral cooperation becomes progressively easier as one moves down the political hierarchy or down the levels of governmental organization. Jealousies and rivalries at the high levels may make cooperation difficult. Thus multisectoral cooperation becomes easier at the local or community

---

Box 5.2 The Education Sector and NCDs

At the level of government, the education sector deals primarily with formal education, usually in institutions. The impact of education is through providing an environment in which the young are socialized into health habits—e.g., avoiding the risk factors for NCDs. But important habits are also inculcated through pedagogy. One example from the Caribbean is a Health and Family Life Education Program, which has the following standard as one of the themes of its curriculum: "Building individual capacity to make healthy choices throughout the life cycle and reduce the risk factors associated with the development of life-style diseases." It has also been shown that health and nutrition education at the primary level can reduce the prevalence of chronic disease risk factors.[a] Formal education of health workers at the tertiary level obviously influences the practice of medicine and affects both individual as well as population health.

---

[a] Commonwealth Secretariat. *Commonwealth Health Ministers' Update 2011*. London: Pro-Brook Publishing Ltd.; 2011, p. 53.

---

levels. It is also claimed that collaboration between sections or departments of sectors is intrinsically easier than through whole-of-sector arrangements. In the context of NCDs, multisectoral action has largely been confined to concomitant action by different levels of government, mandated and driven by a level above sectoral heads (box 5.3).

Facilitating Multisectoral Cooperation through Health Impact Assessment

Health impact assessment (HIA) represents the most widely accepted approach to ensuring effective multisectoral cooperation. It is defined in the 1999 Gothenburg consensus statement as "a combination of procedures, methods, and tools by which a policy, program, or project may be judged as to its potential effects on the health of a population, and the distribution of those effects within the population."[9] It is considered to be the best way of ensuring that health concerns are taken into account in projects/activities that are thought to be outside the health sector.[10] HIA brings public health considerations to the attention of persons and sectors whose main orientation is not health.

It had its conceptual origins in the notion of healthy public policy, which is one of the five key health promotion actions identified in the Ottawa Charter.[11] Healthy public policy is only possible when the health consequences of various

---

Box 5.3 Multisectoral Action for NCDs by Governments

Turkey, Egypt, and Ukraine have recently been successful in implementing multisectoral action for NCD prevention in the area of tobacco control; in each case, action by government agencies outside the health sector has been evident. In Turkey, the Turkish Regulatory Agency for Cigarettes and Alcoholic Beverages was at the forefront.[a] In Ukraine, the Ukrainian Institute of Social Research, the Kiev International Institute of Sociology, the Supreme Rada Committee (the government taxation authority), and the Ukraine State Statistical Office were assisting the parliament with laws that were enacted.[b]

Examples of countries' successful actions to reduce the harmful use of alcohol also illustrate multisectoral action. In Brazil, a new health minister coordinated the creation of an interministerial group to set guidelines for a policy concerning alcohol-related problems. In China, the China Consumers' Association, in addition to the public agencies directly responsible for setting health policies, became involved in the issue.[c] In Vietnam, action on alcohol was the combined result of the Committee for Social Affairs of the National Assembly, the Ministry of Industry and Trade, the Ministry of Finance, the Vietnam Brewers Association, Vietnam's Alcohol Beer Beverage Association, and the International Center for Alcohol Policies.[d] Multisectoral action for salt reduction, of which the United Kingdom offers the most salient example, involved the UK Food Standards Agency, the UK Scientific Advisory Committee on Nutrition, and the Food and Drink Federation in addition to the Department of Health.

---

[a] Yürekli A, Önder Z, Elibol M, Erk N, Cabuk A, Fisunoglu M, Erk SF, Chaloupka FJ. The economics of tobacco and tobacco taxation in Turkey. Paris: International Union Against Tuberculosis and Lung Disease; 2010. www.who.int/tobacco/en_tfi_turkey_report_feb2011.pdf. Accessed June 18, 2012.

[b] Ross HZ, Shariff S, Gilmore A. Economics of Tobacco Taxation in Ukraine. Paris: International Union Against Tuberculosis and Lung Disease; 2009.

[c] Cochrane J, Chen H, Conigrave K, Hao W. Alcohol use in China. *AA*. 38(6):537–542;2006. http://alcalc .oxfordjournals.org/content/38/6/537.full.

[d] Health Strategy and Policy Institute—Ministry of Health. Sharing experiences for the development of the national policy on alcohol-related harm prevention and control. Hanoi: International Center for Alcohol Policies; 2009. www.icap.org/LinkClick.aspx?fileticket=fWekIg%2B2%2Bek%3D&tabid=72. Accessed June 18, 2012.

---

policy options can be identified and there is some clear mechanism for influencing the development of policy such that health consequences are considered and health promoted and protected. Health impact assessment can be regarded as one of the tools of healthy public policy.[12] It has also been influenced by the logic of environmental impact assessment.[13] To the extent that policy formulation in health is quintessentially the function of government, it is obvious that this tool has its most useful application in multisectoral cooperation.

The U.S. Centers for Disease Control and Prevention maintains an extensive bibliography on the use of health impact assessment and its increasing utilization at many different levels of government.[14] According to the CDC, major steps in conducting an HIA include

- Screening (identifying plans, projects, or policies for which an HIA would be useful)
- Scoping (identifying which health effects to consider)
- Assessing risks and benefits (identifying which people may be affected and how they may be affected)
- Developing recommendations (suggesting changes to proposals to promote positive health effects or minimize adverse health effects)
- Reporting (presenting the results to decision makers)
- Monitoring and evaluating (determining the effect of the HIA on the decision)

WHO also provides extensive material on the methodologies and examples of how HIA has been applied in nonhealth sectors such as agriculture, housing, and tourism, among others.[15] Indeed, there is no limit to the possible number of sectors in government that might be involved in determining the health impact assessment of a particular project. It is possible, however, that this powerful tool is more applicable to discrete programs or projects, rather than for ongoing cooperation over a broad field, such as is the case with the whole of another sector's basic functions and responsibilities that affect health.

Intersectoral Cooperation
Antecedents

One can trace the interest in intersectoral cooperation back to the Declaration of Alma-Ata, which defined primary healthcare and specified that it "involves, in addition to the health sector, all related sectors and aspects of national and community development, in particular agriculture, animal husbandry, food, industry, education, housing, public works, communications and other sectors; and demands the coordinated efforts of all those sectors."[16] The declaration referred uniquely to the institutions of government, and the standard requisites for effective primary healthcare were set out as intersectoral cooperation, appropriate technology, and community participation. In the landmark conference by WHO on intersectoral cooperation in Halifax, Canada, in 1997, the definition of "intersectoral action for health" adopted was "A recognized relationship between part or parts of the health sector with part or parts of another sector which has been formed to take action on an issue to achieve health outcomes or intermediate health outcomes in a way that is more effective, efficient or sustainable than could be achieved by the health sector alone."[17] In this definition, the orientation was entirely toward the public sector or the government.

The WHO World Health Report of 2008, "Primary health care: now more than ever" referred to the fact that health figured prominently in the MDGs and this "created the necessary social conditions for the establishment of close alliances beyond the health sector. Thus intersectoral action is back on center stage." However, the emphasis was on cooperation among the sectors of government—the "whole of government" approach—in addressing the major problems to be solved.[18] The WHO Commission on the Social Determinants of Health emphasized the absolute imperative of considering that several sectors beyond health determined the state of individual or population health.[19] In its purpose, the WHO 2008–2013 Action Plan for the Global Strategy for the Prevention and Control of Noncommunicable Diseases speaks to "leading and catalyzing an intersectoral, multilevel response," although it applies the notion of intersectoriality to cooperation between and among parts of government.[20]

Intersectoral Cooperation as Currently Interpreted

More recently, intersectoral cooperation has been restricted to cooperation among the sectors of the state—the government, the private sector or business, and civil society (fig. 5.2). This is referred to in the Political Declaration within the context of the whole-of-society approach. However, some of the actors mentioned in the PD, such as individuals, families, and communities who are critical for the prevention and control of NCDs, do not usually contribute directly in sectoral approaches. Whereas in the case of multisectoral cooperation, we assume that there is a uniformly liberal interest in health matters, this cannot be assumed to exist in the sectors of the state. They have essentially different interests, but the assumption is that their particular skills and assets can be combined to improve health.[21]

The government and its institutions should be concerned with public order and producing public goods. At its disposal are the instruments of legislation, regulation, and taxation through which it can establish conditions for human development and pursue it, given that it is one of the highest societal goals. The market, or the private sector, is concerned with the efficient production of goods and services and has profit as its fundamental raison d'etre. However, the private sector or at least the more enlightened parts of it has always accepted corporate social responsibility and the principle that business in general does well by doing

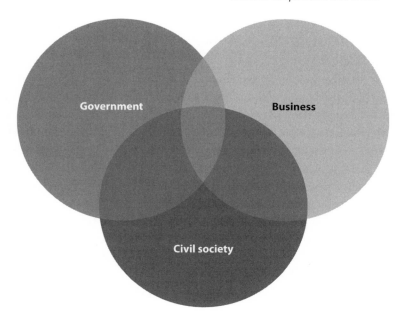

Fig. 5.2. Intersectoral cooperation: the intersection between the three sectors of the state.

good. More recently, the concept of shared value has been put forward, which proposes that the competitiveness of a company and the well-being of its community are mutually dependent and that there is an intimate connection between societal and economic progress.[22]

Civil society is not a monolithic entity. It is composed of multiple types of groups, of which nongovernmental organizations are but one. Its strengths as a sector lie in its ability to respond to different issues of societal importance and mobilize public opinion. The weaknesses intrinsic to its diversity are well known, as is its power to articulate and promote values-driven propositions and be a watchdog to prevent abuse by the government. In many instances it serves as an honest broker between government and the private sector.[23]

One view of intersectoral cooperation is that sectors of society collaborate only when they absolutely have to do so and in other instances, the collaboration is driven by external agents.[24] The success of intersectoral collaboration has been attributed to the following: forging initial agreements, building leadership, building legitimacy, building trust, managing conflict, and planning.[25] All of these factors are important, but perhaps priority might be given to building leadership, building trust, and planning. The leadership usually comes from the government, and one of the difficulties that must be overcome in the initial planning stage is the almost instinctive distrust of the private sector by civil society. This has to be overcome by clearly defining the rules of engagement and establishing the parameters of conflict of interest. It is critical that in matters of public policy, while there may be cooperation in providing the data with which policy can be formed, the actual formation of public policy is the particular and sole responsibility of the government. Other sectors may collaborate in the execution of the policy but never in its formulation.

A less well-tapped mode of engaging private participation for public goals centers on harnessing market forces for regulation. By creating the right policy framework and agreement on a set of norms, an incentive can be created for both quality and the delivery of service.

Modes of Intersectoral Collaboration

Interersectoral cooperation may involve all three sectors, but more frequently it involves only two. Government-NGO relationships are common, especially in situations in which government engages a nonprofit organization to carry out activities that might normally be the responsibility of government. The relationship between the government and the nonprofit may take the form of a principal-agent relationship or be in the nature of a stewardship agreement. In the standard principal-agent relationship, the principal seeks to maximize welfare and the agent seeks to maximize utility. In the stewardship relationship, goal convergence occurs. The two forms are perhaps extremes, and many government-NGO relationships fall somewhere along a continuum between the principal-agent mode and the stewardship arrangement.[26]

Public-private partnerships have emerged as significant mechanisms for achieving global health objectives. They have been described as "relatively institutionalized initiatives, established to address global health problems, in which public and private-for-profit sector organizations have a voice in collective decision making."[27] Their emergence has been due to the complexity of the global health challenges, the recognition that the production of global public goods may be beyond the capacity of the public sector, the need for the speed and agility that characterize the private sector orientation, and the "availability of unprecedented resources, largely precipitated by the Bill and Melinda Gates Foundation."[28] Public-private partnerships are diverse arrangements that bring together actors with varying goals and motivations in the pursuit of similar objectives. The nature of public

---

Box 5.4 Pakistan—Intersectoral Action for NCDs

In Pakistan, an NGO has created a social protection program for health that aims to protect people from catastrophic healthcare costs and medical impoverishment. The program ensures financial access of poor people to essential medicines and treatments for noncommunicable diseases.[a] While the core objective centers on health, the sectors on which this program has drawn for its construct and functioning are almost all outside of the health systems and the health sector. Reliance on m-Health and its user-friendly integration with web-based technology enables efficient processing of requests and monitoring of service delivery. Technology has enabled innovations in donation management that empower the donor to earmark donations and track microtransaction details in real time. Use of technology has been critical in eliminating abuse in targeting and pilferage from the system. This system, entitled Heartfile Health Financing, has strategically leveraged philanthropy as one of the means of financing. Partnership with the Pakistan Poverty Alleviation Fund enables it to tap into resources that are outside of the traditional health system, and through an online interface with Pakistan's National Database Registration Authority, it can access a national poverty database to ascertain patients' eligibility. The program is being integrated with platforms that enable mobile payments. It is reconfiguring its process to comply with central bank regulations so that its current grants module can be expanded, with health loans as an additional feature.

---

[a] Nishtar S, Khalid F, Batool N, et al. Heartfile health financing: striving to achieve health equity in Pakistan. www.who.int/sdhconference/resources/draft_background_paper26_pakistan.pdf. Accessed Dec 2, 2011; Nishtar S, Khalid F, Ikram A, et al. Protecting the poor against health impoverishment in Pakistan: proof of concept of the potential within innovative web and mobile phone technologies. Background Paper to World Health Report, 2010, Health Systems Financing. World Health Organization, 2010. www.who.int /healthsystems/topics/research/55Heartfile_HEF_POC.pdf.

---

health action in NCDs warrants an intersectoral response with partnerships as its key feature. However, it is important to note that of more than one hundred global partnerships on health, not even one is explicitly focused on NCDs.[29] Yet, there are examples in a few countries of public-private frameworks, both for policy as well as implementation of NCD policy.[30]

The burgeoning of new technologies and transformative tools such as m-Health is rapidly changing the inventory of potential collaborators towards multisectoral action. A new emphasis on bottom-of-pyramid technologies, outreach tools, telecommunication connectivity, and innovative means of resource generation is rapidly altering the landscape of actors and potential partners that become relevant in multisectoral action toward achieving NCD prevention and management goals (box 5.4).

Benefits of Sectoral Cooperation

Sectoral cooperation, whether intersectoral or multisectoral, should produce public value. In general, it should produce economies of scale and gains in productivity, especially through reducing duplication. It should result in improved health, particularly at the population level, and it is critical for the prevention and control of NCDs, as indicated in the PD. Cooperation is not without costs, and there is inherent conflict which must be managed. The sectoral approach to addressing the dominant risk factors for NCDs is shown schematically in table 5.1, where we indicate which of the sectors is most likely to be involved.

Governance

Governance presents challenges in all sectoral cooperation. In the case of health, the lead is usually taken by the health sector, which has the capacity to outline the nature of the problem to be addressed with the most precision. The best results are obtained when another sector addresses the nonhealth area that affects health as part of its regular activities and does not have to divert resources from the basic work and concern of the sector; the success of this approach has been pointed out in the case of HIV/AIDS.

There is less need for formal joint agreement in many instances of multisectoral cooperation. The financial sector or the finance minister makes the decision to raise tobacco taxes not only because smoking contributes to disease, but also often for good fiscal reasons. Intersectoral cooperation may be different, as there is usually a need for a more formal agreement describing the responsibility of the relevant partners. In the case of the government-NGO relationship for project execution, this agreement is a formal contract.

Table 5.1   Intersectoral involvement in addressing NCD risk factors

Risk factor	Government	Private sector	Civil society
Tobacco	++++	none	++
Physical inactivity	++	+	+
Harmful use of alcohol	++++	?	++
Unhealthy diet	++	+++	?

Note: Plus signs are an indication of the strength of involvement of the sectors. A question mark indicates that it is questionable whether any involvement exists.

The PD refers to multisectoral action at the global level, which presents a special challenge. Some of the vectors responsible for NCDs cross national borders. The propaganda that promotes smoking and behaviors inimical to health permeate national borders, and the businesses responsible for them are global. In the case of tobacco, there is clearly no cooperation, but a formal treaty—the WHO Framework Convention on Tobacco Control. It may be useful to think of a similar mechanism for some of the other products that are known to be risk factors for NCDs, such as salt. The best possibility for establishing any form of global governance to effect sectoral cooperation with regard to NCDs is through the World Health Organization, which has the constitutional responsibility "to act as the directing and co-coordinating authority on international health work."

Summary

Sectoral interaction is essential in health, particularly for the prevention and control of NCDs, which present a major and growing health problem. Multisectoriality is referenced frequently in the Political Declaration from the UN High-level Meeting on the Prevention and Control of Non-communicable Diseases of September 2011. This chapter makes a clear distinction between multisectoral and intersectoral approaches, setting out the relevant actors in both. Multisectoriality refers essentially to interaction among the administrative agencies of the government, while intersectoriality applies to the interaction among the three main actors of the state: the public sector, the private sector, and civil society. Examples of both forms of sectoral cooperation are given. The modes of effecting multisectoral and intersectoral action are defined and the possible governance mechanism for sectoral cooperation is outlined. The taxonomy proposed here should be of value in establishing the boundaries and responsibilities in sectoral cooperation for the prevention and control of NCDs.

NOTES

1. United Nations General Assembly. Political Declaration of the High-level Meeting of the General Assembly on the Prevention and Control of Non-communicable Diseases A/66/L.1. www.cfr.org/global-health/political-declaration-high-level-meeting-general-assembly-prevention-control-non-communicable-diseases/p25953. Accessed May 12, 2012.

2. World Health Organization. Global status report on non-communicable diseases, 2010. Geneva: WHO; 2010.

3. Bloom DE, Cafiero ET, Jané-Llopis E, et al. The global economic burden of non-communicable diseases. Geneva: World Economic Forum; 2011.

4. World Health Organization. Discussion Paper 1: Effective approaches for strengthening multisectoral action for NCDs. Geneva: World Health Organization; in press.

5. World Health Organization. EB130.R7: Prevention and control of non-communicable diseases: follow-up to the High-level Meeting of the United Nations General Assembly on the Prevention and Control of Non-communicable Diseases, ninth meeting. http://apps.who.int/gb/ebwha/pdf_files/EB130/B130_R7-en.pdf. Accessed June 1, 2012.

6. CARICOM Heads of Government. Declaration of Port-of-Spain: Uniting to Stop the Epidemic of Chronic NCDs. Port-of-Spain: CARICOM Secretariat; September 15, 2007. www.caricom.org/jsp/communications/meetings_statements/declaration_port_of_spain_chronic_ncds.jsp. Accessed May 11, 2012.

7. World Bank. A new instrument to advance development effectiveness: program-for-results financing. Washington, DC: World Bank; 2011. http://documents.worldbank.org/curated/en/2011/12/15590386/new-instrument-advance-development-effectiveness-program-for-results-financing.

8. Bryson, JM, Crosby, BC Stone, MM. The design and implementation of cross-sector collaborations: propositions from the literature. *Public Administration Review* 66:44–55;2006. doi: 10.1111/j.1540-6210.2006.00665.x

9. World Health Organization Regional Office for Europe. 2012. www.euro.who.int/en/what-we-do/health-topics/environmental-health/health-impactassessment.

10. Lock K. Health Impact Assessment. *BMJ* 320:1395–1398;2000.

11. World Health Organization. The Ottawa Charter for Health Promotion. First International Conference on Health Promotion, 21 November 1986. www.who.int/healthpromotion/conferences/previous/ottawa/en/.

12. Kemm J. Health Impact Assessment: a tool for healthy public policy. *Health Promotion International* 16:79–85;2001.

13. Joffe M, Sutcliffe J. Developing policies for a healthy environment. *Health Promotion International* 12:169–173;1997.

14. Centers for Disease Prevention and Control. Health Impact Assessment. www.cdc.gov/healthyplaces/factsheets/Health_Impact_Assessment_factsheet_Final.pdf. Accessed June 18, 2012.

15. World Health Organization. Health Impact assessment. www.who.int/hia/en/. Accessed June 18, 2012.

16. Declaration of Alma-Ata. International Conference on Primary Health Care, Alma-Ata, USSR, 6–12 September, 1978. www.who.int/hpr/NPH/docs/declaration_almaata.pdf.

17. Kreisel W, von Schirnding Y. Intersectoral action for health: a cornerstone for Health for All in the 21st century. *World Health Stat Q.* 1998;51(1):75–78.

18. World Health Organization. World Health Report 2008. Primary health care: now more than ever. Geneva: WHO; 2008.

19. Commission on Social Determinants of Health. Closing the gap in a generation: health equity through action on the social determinants of health. Geneva: WHO, 2008. http://whqlibdoc.who.int/publications/2008/9789241563703_eng.pdf.

20. World Health Organization. 2008–2013 Action Plan for the Global Strategy for the Prevention and Control of Noncommunicable Diseases. Geneva: WHO, 2008.

21. Waddell S, Brown LD. Fostering intersectoral partnering: a guide to promoting cooperation among government, business and civil society actors. Institute for Development Research. *IDR Reports* 13(3)1–26;1997.

22. Porter ME, Kramer MR. Creating shared value. *Harvard Business Review* 89:62–77;2011.

23. Kalegaonkar A, Brown LD. Intersectoral cooperation: lessons for practice. *Institute for Development Reports* 16(2):1–25;2000.

24. Barringer BR, Harrison JS. Walking a tightrope: creating value through interorganizational relationships. *Journal of Management* 26:367–403;2000.

25. Bryson, JM, Crosby, BC, Stone, MM. The design and implementation of cross-sector collaborations: propositions from the literature. *Public Administration Review* 66:44–55;2006. doi: 10.1111/j.1540-6210.2006.00665.x.

26. Caers R, DuBois C, Jegers M, De Gieter S, Schepers C, Pepermans R. Principal-agent relationships on the stewardship-agency axis. *NonProfit Management and Leadership* 17:25–47;2006; Van Slyke DM. Agents or stewards: using theory to understand the government-nonprofit social services contracting relationships. *Journal of Public Admin. Research and Theory* 17(2):157–187;2007.

27. Buse K, Harmer A. Seven habits of highly effective global health partnerships: practice and potential. *Soc Sci Med* 64:259–271;2007.

28. Buse K, Tanaka S. Global public-private health partnerships: lessons learned from ten years of experience and evaluation. *International Dental Journal* 61(Suppl. 2):2–10;2011.

29. Gostin L. Meeting the survival needs of the world's least healthy people: a proposed model for global health governance. *JAMA* 298:225–228;2007; Magnusson RS. Rethinking global health challenges: towards a "global compact" for reducing the burden of chronic disease. *Public Health* 123:265–274;2009; Nishtar S. Time for a global partnership on non-communicable diseases. *Lancet* 370:1887–1888;2007.

30. Nishtar S, Bile KM, Ahmed A, Faruqui AMA, Mirza Z, Shera S, et al. Process, rationale, and interventions of Pakistan's National Action Plan on Chronic Diseases. *Prev Chronic Dis.* 3(1):A14;Jan 2006. Epub Dec 15, 2005.

The Developing World and the Challenge of Noncommunicable Diseases

Stuart Gilmour and Kenji Shibuya

The global health community is marshaling its resources and resolve to take on the challenge of noncommunicable diseases in the developing world. There is good cause to be optimistic, given the tremendous progress that has already been made throughout the world in dealing with infectious diseases. That effort has generated thousands of new institutions, new programs, and new attitudes toward the gap in healthcare between the developed and the developing nations. Millions of lives have been extended and improved through prevention and treatment. Those programs are far from completed and will continue through the rest of this century and beyond, in part to deal with the growing problem of drug-resistant infections. Nevertheless, the major focus of global healthcare is now shifting decisively toward the tremendous and growing burden of noncommunicable diseases in all regions of the world.

The rationale for this transition is embodied in the stark figures on morbidity and mortality, figures that all of the authors in this volume have touched upon, either directly or indirectly. The noncommunicable disease epidemic currently looms as the biggest threat to global health: two-thirds of all deaths are due to NCDs, and the newest global burden of disease (GBD 2010) study supports an invigorated international effort to combat noncommunicable diseases and prevent premature deaths and years lived with disability.[1] Globally, longer life expectancy with increasing disabilities brings with it significant health financing and cost containment issues that cannot be avoided.[2] So too do the changes in health behavior that occur alongside increased incomes and leisure time. This leaves many of the developing nations facing the double burden of campaigning against infectious disease while they muster their health systems to counter noncommunicable diseases.[3] They are also dealing with the demands of health financing reform and the drive to universal health coverage (UHC),[4] a movement that threatens to be derailed by the formidable cost burden that the NCD epidemic presents to their fragile health financing systems.[5] There is, in brief, ample evidence to support a negative prognosis for the global NCD campaign.

All of the authors in this book remain optimistic, however, and we believe their positions are fully justified. The response to the NCD epidemic is still in an early stage of development as a global healthcare initiative. General statements of concern have prompted new thought on the issue and helped focus worldwide attention on what needs to be done to counter the epidemic in the developing world. The importance of responding to this challenge has been clearly recognized,[6] and after the UN General Assembly made its declaration on NCDs,[7] scholars, international public health officials, and national leaders launched debate over the specific policy responses called for by the epidemic. Health system strengthening, intersectorality, public-private partnerships, and new approaches to primary care have all been discussed globally. It is thus timely to publish this book in light of the GBD 2010 study. Framed by the latest, most robust research, the chapters presented here get into the nitty-gritty of what needs to be done to build on the common body of policy ideas. The authors have begun the task of pointing to the new measures that will be needed while they also provide reminders that though the global health context may change, many of the crucial elements of the policy response remain constant.

Making Full Use of Existing Knowledge

Though the topics covered in this collection are diverse, they share a number of themes. The chapters certainly cover a broad range of topics: pharmaceutical regulation and distribution (chapter 1); improved investment in and management of pharmaceutical supply and logistic systems (chapter 2); lessons for NCD policy from the HIV/AIDS policy experience (chapter 3); the reorientation of primary care in the era of NCDs (chapter 4); and proposals for enhancing sectoral collaboration in the battle against NCDs (chapter 5). One of the central themes that emerges is the importance of more effectively implementing existing knowledge about best practice in health policy. This is not to denigrate the need for new research results brought out in a timely manner, but we recognize that much has been learned—from failures as well as successes—and that the readily available information should be used in creative ways. Effective health policy does not necessarily require more or better resources but can be achieved by better and more effective implementation of what is already known. Mattke (chapter 3) shows, for instance, how the first stages of the changes away from an infectious disease focus had to be at the clinical level to combat HIV/AIDS effectively; this is knowledge hard earned and valuable to the NCD campaign. Mattke's studies also indicate that decisive changes—whether at the clinical, agency, or health system level—do not necessarily require new research or technology, but rest primarily on better, more intelligent, and integrated implementation of existing techniques that are backed up by intersectoral cooperation and good governance.

Improving Governance

Governance issues will clearly be of central importance in health system reorientation to tackle NCDs. In the long term, certain specific improvements in governance at both the country and global levels will be essential. The challenges of pharmaceutical regulation and distribution, particularly, show that now more than ever before, governance needs to be at the center of the efforts to ensure that all agents in the health sector at all levels are more accountable, more responsive, and better able to provide safe and affordable care in developing nations. The sections of this book (chapters 1 and 2) on potential innovations in pharmaceutical regulation and delivery systems describe the benefits that can accrue to the whole health system from well-understood improvements in diagnostic techniques and pharmaceutical regulation in the developing world. In many societies, major health gains can flow directly from institutional reforms and coordinated control measures in medicine distribution systems.

Central to the governance program will be an emphasis on improved monitoring. Again, this effort can build on existing technologies and well-understood policies in global healthcare. Smith and Yadav (chapter 2) and White-Guay (chapter 1) describe with care the importance of performance monitoring in improving the response to NCDs at all levels of society. Sound information will provide a base for improved governance and accountability; it will be an essential tool for implementing the latest policy developments intelligently and early. Performance monitoring for NCDs demands a broad suite of tools, implemented at all levels, from the global to the local. At the global level, the GBD project promises to offer more support to country-level research to inform priority setting and thus provide a new level of accountability for global health policy. This should make a substantial difference in the ability to monitor national trends in the burden of key diseases[8] and is particularly important in the context of the new processes to be implemented after the expiration of the Millennium Development Goals. At the national and subnational level, monitoring of institutions such as pharmaceutical regulators, private organizations, and local health authorities promises to improve prescribing practice to reduce costs, increase efficiency, and deliver better health outcomes.[9]

Although many practical and theoretical problems in performance monitoring will remain, recent innovations in the intelligent management of health data offer hope: the growth of digital medical record systems and the concomitant ability to merge medical information from disparate sources and health networks;[10] improved information management and retrieval systems, plus improvements in data mining and machine learning to enable better and more innovative uses of data;[11] and advances in social marketing and personalized technology, such as virtual health networks and personalized health messages on cell phones or social networks, are all ways to use existing health systems to improve both our understanding of barriers to improved health quality and our institutional and individual response to them. In terms of global, regional, and national efforts, and in the drive toward UHC systems that offer effective, low-cost, equitable care, performance monitoring will be an essential tool, and nowhere will it need to be more advanced than in the management of NCDs.

Intersectoral Coordination and Collaboration

Each step forward will call for increased coordination and collaboration in responding to the complex health challenges of NCDs. Reorientation of health services and systems—from the national to the clinic level—was a key to success in the battle against HIV/AIDS, enabling a transformation from relatively narrow clinically focused models of healthcare delivery to multidisciplinary teams capable of responding to and implementing the latest evidence about best practice in

HIV prevention and treatment. Unlike HIV/AIDS, noncommunicable diseases have multifaceted causes and present very complex medical challenges: they call for advances in clinical practice and a new level of performance in the ability to harmonize public health and treatment goals in an environment of rapidly changing evidence for the best interventions.

Developing health policy that will be able to meet these challenges will require responses from a wide cross-section of civil society, and coordinating and implementing these responses will demand the same cross-society commitment and collaborations that characterized the response to HIV/AIDS. Kruk et al. (chapter 4) describe the possibilities for a more responsive, multidisciplinary primary health system capable of managing the challenges of NCDs.

The threat of NCDs thus offers an opportunity to revolutionize health systems in developing nations, to move them beyond their current infectious disease focus, and to enable them to deliver a much broader range of effective and efficient health service interventions. For every such opportunity in health service reform there is a corresponding risk of failure; and failure at this point could doom the health systems in many of the developing nations to excessive costs and a great number of dissatisfied patients. The need is clearly for the type of "leap-frog" innovations in developing countries that would also benefit the ongoing health system reforms in developed countries. As Alleyne and Nishtar indicate in chapter 5, a truly effective cooperative framework will require a shift away from narrow concepts of *multisectoral* (interagency) cooperation to a broader *intersectoral* model, based on cooperation between larger sectors of civil society, including government, the private sector, and community actors. In their chapter, we see the breadth of the challenge and the great promise for further reform that NCDs present.

Enhanced Primary Care

No subject touched on in this book is more important than primary care. Indeed, all of the reforms will ultimately turn on the ability to improve primary care facilities for NCDs. It is appropriate in this context that Kruk, Nigenda, and Knaul focus on the opportunities presented by reorientation of primary health care systems. As they point out in chapter 4, primary care services offer the ideal setting in which to tackle the challenges of early diagnosis and prevention of NCDs, routine disease management, health education, and integrated disease care. Through these services, in turn, health systems can hope to reduce the costs associated with chronic diseases.[12] Early diagnosis and quality primary care management can also reduce costs and improve health outcomes.[13] However, any such health service reorientation will be ineffective without a move to universal health coverage, reorientation of existing infectious disease–focused systems toward a vision of health management and primary prevention, and a focus on equity and health access for all.[14] Research in developed nations shows that without proper oversight and engagement, primary care will not necessarily yield public health gains and may even increase inequities.[15] Reorientation of health systems toward primary care therefore needs to be done with awareness of the limitations and benefits of this systemic approach; primary care is not a panacea that can be utilized without the elements of strong governance, coordination, and good systems management.

A New Stakeholder Vision

In the area of sustainability and long-term viability, NCDs offer the greatest challenges (see chapter 5). In their efforts to achieve the UN goals, reformers need to remain constantly aware of the threat to the long-term sustainability of health financing systems that NCDs represent. Savedoff et al. summarized features common to many countries in the process of achieving UHC, including attention to economic growth, demographics, modern technology, the politics of healthcare, and health spending patterns.[16] This complex array of factors is further confounded by growing difficulties in global health leadership, diverging priorities, and global economic uncertainties. Obviously, the previously common donor-driven approach to health-related MDGs may not be ideal for tackling NCDs, and a new global health partnership and business model may be needed to address systemic issues, quality of care, and health financing. Here the stakeholders should be expanded from governments, bilateral organizations, and multilateral organizations to incorporate the private sector, civil society, and foundations. The role of the global health community would then shift from simply the provision of financial resources and project implementation to counseling and advising strategies and to developing innovative approaches and exercising convening powers.

The shift in the global burden of disease from communicable to noncommunicable disease represents a huge transformation in the way health systems have to work and presents a new set of issues. With these challenges come opportunities to revolutionize the action of health systems and their ability to collaborate with, and engage, a broad range of sectors of society. The chapters in this book probe the problems and opportunities that lie ahead in the reorientation of health systems to focus on the new health threats that have emerged as infectious diseases have declined. We firmly believe that reorientation will take place gradually and unevenly but decisively in the long term.

The chapters in this book provide specific steps forward as the developed and developing nations search for a new common approach to the NCD epidemic. As the global health policy community moves to implement the WHO's new agenda for UHC and responds to the growing threat to sustainability posed by the epidemic of NCDs, concrete policy goals and actions are needed to define a new healthcare framework. We believe that progress should involve the following four key policies:

1. *Multisectoral commitment*: Different societies have different patterns of stakeholder engagement with the goal of dealing effectively with NCDs; there will be various patterns of resistance[17] to change; and policy makers need to engage, across sectors, those stakeholders with the strongest commitment to reform. For disparate societies at differing stages of progress, balanced and gradual goals need to be set to ensure bipartisanship and grassroots support. Effective multisectoral cooperation in the developed and the developing countries will be crucial to the achievement of a new institutional and policy base for coping with the NCD epidemic.

2. *Improvements in performance monitoring*: Performance monitoring is essential not only to understanding what works and what does not but to understanding the future burden of disease that health systems will face and to managing the cost and resource issues that NCDs present to health finance planning.[18] For NCDs, performance monitoring means not only measuring disease end states and their related health service burden but also the success of intermediate health agencies—especially primary care services—in routine management of NCDs, maintaining patient quality of life, and constraining costs. Health financing agencies (private or public) will need to push to merge data from primary and secondary care facilities and pharmaceutical dispensers, to understand how both prescribing practice and routine disease management will affect long-term health care costs and hospital utilization. Performance monitoring needs to move beyond the observation of disease end-states

to monitoring the efficiency and cost of disease management processes. The use of large data sets and modern methods of data mining, predictive modeling to reduce hospital admissions, and sophisticated algorithms for personalizing medicine should be implemented where the data are available. Data analysis and reporting is not enough in itself, however, and successful performance monitoring requires improved feedback mechanisms, both through engagement of the medical community in ongoing quality improvement processes and through the use of innovative telemedicine and social marketing processes to push findings on preventive medicine outside of the health system, to individuals and stakeholders. These changes will be particularly challenging for health systems in developing nations, where data collections are still in development and reporting systems weak or fragmented.

3. *Engagement of nontraditional sectors with health*: Intersectoral cooperation demands the engagement of agencies and organizations traditionally considered outside the boundaries of the health sector: corporations, community groups, religious organizations, and unions can all play a role in intersectoral cooperation and can all form their own partnerships with health agencies. These partnerships should engage nonhealth sector actors at a deeper level than in their traditional role as donors: they need to be able to take a proactive role in setting and implementing the health agenda. In engaging these nontraditional actors, the global health community will have to take a stronger role in convening and coordinating initiatives from outside the traditional health sector and working to align their goals with the NCD and UHC agendas. Global health programs directed at the risk factors for NCDs should operate outside of a narrow health framework, targeting work practices, consumption habits, transportation, and leisure activities; innovative programs in all of these areas will require the active cooperation of the main stakeholders in those sectors. Engagement of those stakeholders will require new cross-community, and increasingly cross-national, partnerships.

4. *Modernization of primary care*: The institutions of greatest importance to all of these reforms will be those involved with primary care. Primary care is the layer of the health sector best suited to the prevention and management of NCDs and is also the best setting for

innovative multidisciplinary systems that can improve patient well-being and reduce costs (see chapter 4). However, some countries are still developing a primary care framework or have a primary care system focused only on infectious diseases. Primary care systems need to be modernized to ensure that they are responsive to patient needs, play a strong role in public health programs, have the resources for proper management of NCDs, and have the ability to target risk factors for NCDs. At the health system level, this means enhancing support for early diagnosis of disease and structuring payment systems to ensure that primary care physicians and nurse practitioners have the time and opportunity to offer prevention services and public health interventions; this will enable development of coordinated care plans rather than simply a focus on disease symptoms at the point of care. As shown in the preceding chapters, a wide range of models for successful primary care management of NCDs exists and can be leveraged by national and local health agencies to ensure that the most effective and appropriate primary care systems are in place.

The analysis of the NCD crisis presented here rightfully focuses on the importance of multisectoral and intersectoral cooperation, good governance, innovation in the application of existing knowledge, and reformed primary care as key to successfully overcoming the NCD challenge. We have learned many lessons from past successes against existing health problems, such as HIV/AIDS. Now the global health community needs to adapt these lessons to the new problems faced in the developing nations. The reforms that lie ahead will require significant changes in policy and practice. New stakeholders from a wider community need to be found and engaged, which will require new modes of building and maintaining partnerships. If health policy makers can adapt to these new partnerships, innovations, and community engagements, then the challenge of NCDs can also be transformed into an opportunity to improve the equity, efficiency, and responsiveness of health systems for the betterment of all of society.

NOTES

This work was supported by a Ministry of Health, Labour and Welfare Grant (grant name: *chikyu-kibo-ippan* 007) and a Ministry of Education, Culture, Sports,

Science and Technology grant (grant number 25253051). The funders had no influence over the content or writing of this work.

1. Murray CJL, Vos T, Lozano R, Naghavi M, Flaxman AD, Michaud C, et al. Disability-adjusted life years (DALYs) for 291 diseases and injuries in 21 regions, 1990–2010: a systematic analysis for the Global Burden of Disease Study 2010. *Lancet*. 2012;380(9859):2197–223; Lozano R, Naghavi M, Foreman K, Lim S, Shibuya K, Aboyans V, et al. Global and regional mortality from 235 causes of death for 20 age groups in 1990 and 2010: a systematic analysis for the Global Burden of Disease Study 2010. *Lancet*. 2012;380(9859):2095–128.

2. Anderson GF. Medicare and chronic conditions. *New England Journal of Medicine*. 2005;353(3):305–9.

3. Yach D, Hawkes C, Gould C, Hofman K. The global burden of chronic diseases: overcoming impediments to prevention and control. *Journal of the American Medical Association*. 2004;291(21):2616–22.

4. Sachs JD. Achieving universal health coverage in low-income settings. *Lancet*. 2012;380(9845):944–7; Rodin J, de Ferranti D. Universal health coverage: the third global health transition? *Lancet*. 2012;380(9845):861–2.

5. Samb B, Desai N, Nishtar S, Mendis S, Bekedam H, Wright A, et al. Prevention and management of chronic disease: a litmus test for health-systems strengthening in low-income and middle-income countries. *Lancet*. 2010;376(9754):1785–97.

6. World Health Organization. 2008–2013 Action Plan for the Global Strategy for the Prevention and Control of Noncommunicable Diseases. Geneva: WHO; 2008.

7. World Health Organization. Political Declaration of the High-level Meeting of the General Assembly on the Prevention and Control of Non-communicable Diseases. New York: United Nations; 2011.

8. Chan M. From new estimates to better data. *Lancet*. 2012;380(9859):2054.

9. Fineberg HV. A successful and sustainable health system—how to get there from here. *New England Journal of Medicine*. 2012;366(11):1020–7.

10. Pagliari C, Detmer D, Singleton P. Potential of electronic personal health records. *BMJ*. 2007;335(7615):330–3.

11. Jha AK, Perlin JB, Kizer KW, Dudley RA. Effect of the transformation of the veterans affairs health care system on the quality of care. *New England Journal of Medicine*. 2003;348(22):2218–27; Lakhani A, Coles J, Eayres D, Spence C, Rachet B. Creative use of existing clinical and health outcomes data to assess NHS performance in England: Part 1—performance indicators closely linked to clinical care. *British Medical Journal*. 2005;330(7505):1426–31.

12. Bodenheimer T, Berry-Millett R. Follow the money—controlling expenditures by improving care for patients needing costly services. *New England Journal of Medicine*. 2009;361(16):1521–3.

13. Boult C, Wieland G. Comprehensive primary care for older patients with multiple chronic conditions: "nobody rushes you through." *Journal of the American Medical Association*. 2010;304(17):1936–43.

14. Geneau R, Stuckler D, Stachenko S, McKee M, Ebrahim S, Basu S, et al. Raising the priority of preventing chronic diseases: a political process. *Lancet.* 2010;376(9753):1689–98.

15. Dixon A, Khachatryan A, Gilmour S. Does general practice reduce health inequalities? Analysis of quality and outcomes framework data. *European Journal of Public Health.* 2012;22(1):9–13; McBride D, Hardoon S, Walters K, Gilmour S, Raine R. Explaining variation in referral from primary to secondary care: cohort study. *British Medical Journal.* 2010;341:c6267.

16. Savedoff WD, de Ferranti D, Smith AL, Fan V. Political and economic aspects of the transition to universal health coverage. *Lancet.* 2012;380(9845):924–32.

17. Ibid.

18. Alwan A, Maclean DR, Riley LM, d'Espaignet ET, Mathers CD, Stevens GA, et al. Monitoring and surveillance of chronic non-communicable diseases: progress and capacity in high-burden countries. *Lancet.* 2010;376(9755):1861–8.

Index